Atlas of Minimally Invasive Facelift

Jose Maria Serra-Renom
Jose Maria Serra-Mestre

Atlas of Minimally Invasive Facelift

Facial Rejuvenation with Volumetric Lipofilling

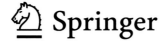

Springer

Jose Maria Serra-Renom
Universitat International de Catalunya
Hospital Quirón Barcelona
Department of Plastic, Reconstructive, and
Aesthetic Surgery
Barcelona
Spain

Jose Maria Serra-Mestre
Universitat International de Catalunya
Hospital Quirón Barcelona
Department of Plastic, Reconstructive, and
Aesthetic Surgery
Barcelona
Spain

ISBN 978-3-319-33016-7   ISBN 978-3-319-33018-1   (eBook)
DOI 10.1007/978-3-319-33018-1

Library of Congress Control Number: 2016945175

Printed on acid-free paper

This Springer imprint is published by Springer Nature
The registered company is Springer International Publishing AG Switzerland

To Rosalia, mother and wife.
José Maria Serra-Renom

This book is dedicated to my family; to my friend and mentor Prof. Francesco D'Andrea, who has been an inspiration and an unflagging support through the years; and to Dr. Oren Tepper, for sharing his thoughts and valuable expertise in craniofacial surgery and surgical planning using 3D-imaging and 3D-printing technologies.
José Maria Serra-Mestre

Preface

Our body image is the dynamic perception we have of our body. Alterations to our body image, either congenital or acquired over a lifetime, can cause significant distress. Like the disproportionate development of the nose or ears during puberty, the changes in tissues during aging can cause considerable suffering for some people, even though aging in itself is a good thing.

In the facial region, our improved understanding of the volumetric changes in fat and bone tissue that occur with the passage of time has revolutionized our conception of facial rejuvenation. The aim today is not just to correct sagging facial tissue but also to restore the volume lost in particular areas in order to reconstruct a rejuvenated facial contour and to improve tissue quality. In many cases, fat and its stromal vascular fraction are key components of treatment.

The clinical applications of adipose tissue have undergone a remarkable expansion in recent years. Although liposuction had been in use for some time, its development in the 1980s and the systematization of the atraumatic protocol developed by Dr. Coleman in the 1990s vastly improved the results obtained, especially in terms of fat graft survival. In recent years, there has been a growing trend toward the use of cannulas of ever-smaller diameter, and even needles at the more superficial level, which have allowed notable improvements in cases of fine remodeling. The range of sizes of fat grafts is particularly important in the facial region in order to prevent irregularities.

For their part, facelift techniques have evolved significantly and are now able to avoid the signs associated with the classical approaches. They now involve moderate dissection of tissues to allow fat grafting in the central areas of the face. There is also a growing tendency toward a combination of techniques, making it possible to achieve results that are both more natural and more complete.

The *Atlas of Minimally Invasive Facelift: Facial Rejuvenation with Volumetric Lipofilling* is a comprehensive description of all the current techniques and applications of facial fat grafting and facelift.

The first section presents the different theories of aging and the effect of the passing of time on different tissues of the facial region. We also discuss the current state of knowledge on fat injection and the possible complications.

The second section, which is organized topographically, provides surgeons with the information needed to successfully accomplish volumetric rejuvenation in the various areas in which we use fat in the facial region, as well as a step-by-step description of the main minimally invasive facelift techniques. This section has been written as clearly and straightforwardly as possible and is supported by a set of very precise illustrations. We hope that this atlas, with its detailed depictions of all the stages involved, will show surgeons the mode and the plane of the injections in each area and will also indicate when superficial and deep injections should be combined.

In the final chapter, we present some clinical cases to illustrate the techniques discussed in the previous sections.

Barcelona, Spain

Jose Maria Serra-Renom
Jose Maria Serra-Mestre

Acknowledgments

The authors would like to express their appreciation to Roser Torres and Michael Maudsley for their assistance during the preparation of this book and to all the members of the Anesthesia Team, for taking care of the patients during the procedures.

Also a special consideration is given to the many plastic surgeons who have contributed their time and research to better understand the process of facial aging and fat grafting: Drs. Coleman, Rohrich, Tonnard, Jelks, Pessa, Mendelson, Longacker, Fontdevila, Benito, Beut, Vinyals, Martí, Khouri, Cervelli, and Mojallal, among others.

Contents

Part I

General Principles

Theories of Facial Aging: Gravitational Versus Volumetric

The aging of the facial region is a continuous, dynamic process in which different tissues are involved. The phenotype of an aging face is not just the product of isolated changes in different tissue planes revealed by anatomic and radiologic studies such as bone remodeling, tissue descent secondary to gravity, attenuation of the retaining facial ligaments, atrophy of fat compartments, and structural and functional impairments in different layers of the skin; it is also the result of the interaction among all these factors.

Precisely because facial aging is caused by a combination of causes and mechanisms of action on a very wide range of tissues in which modifications at one plane affect all the others, there is no one isolated theory that can provide a clinical understanding of its development. Probably the best way to understand it is to link together the different theories that have been put forward to explain these changes.

In this chapter we will not assess the changes at the molecular or cellular level [1] that occur with the passage of time or the effects of environmental factors on tissues such as solar radiation, unhealthy lifestyles, and smoking [2, 3], which clearly have a role to play in the physiologic and functional deterioration of the different structures. Rather, we focus on the main theories which, from a clinical point of view, help to explain the development of the aged face over time and the suitability of each surgical technique in specific cases.

Over the years many theories have been put forward to try to explain facial aging from a clinical perspective. Broadly speaking, they can be summarized under two headings: the gravitational theory and the volumetric theory, which include the model of pseudoptosis.

The gravitational theory emerged during the 1990s, after the description by Furnas [4] of osseocutaneous and musculocutaneous fibrous condensations that help to stabilize and support the different structures of the facial region. This theory identifies the increased laxity of the facial retaining ligaments and the loss of their ability to support facial soft tissue

as the main cause of the face's vertical descent, including excessive sagging and the appearance of folds or creases.

Authors like Stuzin et al. [5] or later Mendelson [6–8] studied these multilinked fibrous ligaments and the facial spaces in depth. They posited that continuous muscle activity causing the stretching of the facial ligaments, together with the intrinsic changes typical of aging, is probably responsible for the weakness and elongation of this ligamentous support, leading to subsequent tissue ptosis.

In accordance with this gravitational theory, lifting techniques were introduced involving a wide dissection of the superficial musculoaponeurotic system (SMAS) [9] in order to reach the retaining ligaments and section them and then to reposition the tissues. In our view, when a ligament is elongated, this procedure is unnecessary. As well as being preferable from the point of view of safety, avoiding wide dissections of the SMAS preserves the system's vascularization, prevents its atrophy, and does not leave two scar planes, one subcutaneous and the other sub-SMAS. It also does not affect the possibility of injecting fat [10].

The gravitational theory was generally accepted until the early 2000s, when observational studies [11, 12] began to identify differences in behavior between different facial regions. It was proposed that the changes in the facial region may not be caused only by a vertical descent and ptosis of the tissues but also by a redistribution of volumes between the soft tissue and facial skeleton of the different subunits of the face.

Indeed, analyzing volumetric changes in the aging midface using high-resolution magnetic resonance imaging, Gosain et al. [13] noted a generalized redistribution of fat and a selective hypertrophy of the upper portion of the surface fat pad in older patients. His group suggested that ptosis alone does not account for the changes observed in the aging midface. Lambros [12], in a comparison of photographs of 83 patients at different stages in their lives, noted that the vast majority of skin landmarks in the periorbital and midface and the lid-cheek position did not descend over time. This author

© Springer International Publishing Switzerland 2016
J.M. Serra-Renom, J.M. Serra-Mestre, *Atlas of Minimally Invasive Facelift*, DOI 10.1007/978-3-319-33018-1_1

hypothesized that the vertical descent of the skin and subcutaneous tissue was not a major component of the midfacial aging process; if the face actually sagged, one would expect to see downward migration of skin landmarks.

For many years, facial fat was considered a confluent mass divided into a superficial plane and a deep plane in relation to the SMAS and the muscles of facial expression. Later, Macchi et al. [14, 15] and Raskin and Latrenta [16] proposed that the distinction between superficial and deep planes was insufficient and that more divisions should be made. It was the study by Rohrich and Pessa [17] that provided anatomic evidence to support the new volumetric theory. These authors demonstrated the compartmentalization of facial fat into different units or compartments by means of connective tissue membranes in both the superficial and the deep planes. In 2012, analyzing CT images, Gierloff et al. [18] observed an inferior migration of the midfacial fat compartments and an inferior volume shift within the compartments during aging, concluding that distinct compartment-specific changes contribute to the aged appearance of the face.

In parallel to this understanding of the redistribution of volumes in the different fat compartments of the facial region with aging, some radiologic studies also showed a resorption and recession in specific locations in the facial skeleton [19], which are described in more detail in Chap. 2. As in the case of the atrophy of the deep fat compartments, these changes in the facial skeleton not only lead to a selective loss of projection in specific areas but reduce the support for the more superficial soft tissue and fat compartments and cause a certain degree of remodeling. In addition, bone recession may alter the position of the attachments of facial muscles and ligaments through the periosteum, which presents a slight backward displacement.

This loss of support caused by volumetric changes in deep structures has given rise to the model of pseudoptosis [20] inside the volumetric theory. This model is the result of the clinical observation that restoring and giving volume in the deep compartments of the malar region not only corrects the negative vector (the projection of the malar region that remains in front of the corneal surface when seen in profile) but also improves other areas such as the nasolabial folds.

The theory of pseudoptosis suggests that selective deflation of the deep fat pads with age leads to a loss of support and the descent of the overlying superficial fat, thereby contributing to the ptotic appearance of the aging face.

The effect is like that created by inflating or deflating a balloon. When full of volume, the superficial compartments located between the deep compartments and the skin remain in position. When the deep compartments lose volume, the support is lost, and the superficial compartments are no longer impacted on the dermis; when this volume is lost, the tissue manifests ptosis.

The evolution of these two theories of facial aging, the gravitational and volumetric, shows why there is a need not

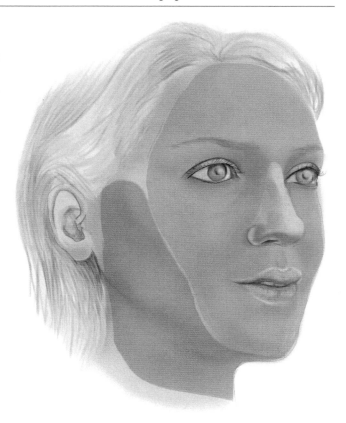

Fig. 1.1 Face and neck rejuvenation techniques need to correct sagging in the peripheral areas of the face using facelift techniques (*red*) but also to reverse the atrophy and redistribute volume in the central regions of the face (*green*)

only to correct sagging in the peripheral areas of the face and neck using facelift techniques but also to reverse the atrophy and redistribute volume in the central regions of the face—which, after all, are the most visible areas [21, 22].

Therefore, to obtain the most natural-looking results possible, it is necessary to use techniques that rejuvenate both the peripheral and the central areas of the face, complementing conventional approaches with procedures to provide volume at the points where it has been lost. Our aim is to reconstruct a rejuvenated facial contour, not just to correct excess skin laxity (Fig. 1.1).

References

1. Makrantonaki E, Zouboulis CC. Molecular mechanisms of skin aging: state of the art. Ann N Y Acad Sci. 2007;1119:40–50.
2. Rexbye H, Petersen I, Johansens M, Klitkou L, Jeune B, Christensen K. Influence of environmental factors on facial ageing. Age Ageing. 2006;35:110–5.
3. Guyuron B, Rowe DJ, Weinfeld AB, Eshraghi Y, Fathi A, Lamphongsai S. Factors contributing to the facial aging of identical twins. Plast Reconstr Surg. 2009;123:1321–31.
4. Furnas DW. The retaining ligaments of the cheek. Plast Reconstr Surg. 1989;83:11–6.

5. Stuzin JM, Baker TJ, Gordon HL. The relationship of the superficial and deep facial fascias: relevance to rhytidectomy and aging. Plast Reconstr Surg. 1992;89:441–9; discussion 450–1.

6. Mendelson BC, Jacobson SR. Surgical anatomy of the midcheek: facial layers, spaces, and the midcheek segments. Clin Plast Surg. 2008;35:395–404.

7. Mendelson BC, Muzaffar AR, Adams Jr WP. Surgical anatomy of the midcheek and malar mounds. Plast Reconstr Surg. 2002;110:885–96.

8. Mendelson BC. Surgery of the superficial musculoaponeurotic system: principles of release, vectors, and fixation. Plast Reconstr Surg. 2001;107:1545–52.

9. Mitz V, Peyronie M. The superficial musculo-aponeurotic system (SMAS) in the parotid and cheek area. Plast Reconstr Surg. 1976;58:80–8.

10. Serra-Renom JM, Diéguez JM, Yoon T. Inferiorly pedicled tongue-shaped SMAS flap transposed to the mastoid to improve the nasolabial fold and jowls and enhance neck contouring during face-lift surgery. Plast Reconstr Surg. 2008;121:298–304.

11. Donofrio LM. Fat distribution: a morphologic study of the aging face. Dermatol Surg. 2000;26:1107–12.

12. Lambros V. Observations on periorbital and midface aging. Plast Reconstr Surg. 2007;120:1367–76; discussion 1377.

13. Gosain AK, Klein MH, Sudhakar PV. A volumetric analysis of soft-tissue changes in the aging midface using high-resolution MRI: implications for facial rejuvenation. Plast Reconstr Surg. 2005;115:1143–52; discussion 1153–5.

14. Macchi V, Tiengo C, Porzionato A, Stecco C, Galli S, Vigato E, et al. Anatomo-radiological study of the superficial musculo-aponeurotic system of the face. Ital J Anat Embryol. 2007;112:247–53.

15. Macchi V, Tiengo C, Porzionato A, Stecco C, Vigato E, Parenti A, et al. Histotopographic study of the fibroadipose connective cheek system. Cells Tissues Organs. 2010;191:47–56.

16. Raskin E, Latrenta GS. Why do we age in our cheeks? Aesthet Surg J. 2007;27:19–28.

17. Rohrich RJ, Pessa JE. The fat compartments of the face: anatomy and clinical implications for cosmetic surgery. Plast Reconstr Surg. 2007;119:2219–27; discussion 2228–31.

18. Gierloff M, Stöhring C, Buder T, Wiltfang J. The subcutaneous fat compartments in relation to aesthetically important facial folds and rhytides. J Plast Reconstr Aesthet Surg. 2012;65:1292–7.

19. Mendelson B, Wong CH. Changes in the facial skeleton with aging: implications and clinical applications in facial rejuvenation. Aesthetic Plast Surg. 2012;36:753–60.

20. Rohrich RJ, Pessa JE, Ristow B. The youthful cheek and the deep medial fat compartment. Plast Reconstr Surg. 2008;121:2107–12.

21. Serra-Renom JM, Serra-Mestre JM. Periorbital rejuvenation to improve the negative vector with blepharoplasty and fat grafting in the malar area. Ophthal Plast Reconstr Surg. 2011;27:442–6.

22. Rohrich RJ, Ghavami A, Constantine FC, Unger J, Mojallal A. Lift-and-fill face lift: integrating the fat compartments. Plast Reconstr Surg. 2014;133:756e–67.

The Anatomic Basis of Facial Aging and Facial Rejuvenation Techniques

As we noted in the previous chapter, it is difficult to present a theory that encompasses all the changes that occur in the aging face. The different mechanisms causing these changes in each of the tissue planes are not yet known. However, the results of anatomic and radiologic studies have shown that it is a problem involving gravitational factors, the distention of supporting structures, changes in volume owing to bone resorption, and especially soft tissue atrophy and redistribution. In addition to these factors is the combination of different genetic factors and biochemical changes, which means that not everyone ages in the same way. The following summary enumerates the most significant changes that occur in the aging face.

2.1 The Skin

The skin is probably the plane that is most exposed to changes caused by aging. It is susceptible to chronic damage from free radicals derived from exposure to sunlight [1, 2] and from environmental factors such as smoking, nutrition, and pollution [3]. It is also influenced by volumetric changes that occur in the deep planes, both in soft tissue and bone.

In addition to these external factors, the skin itself also shows structural and functional changes in its secondary strata caused by a series of intrinsic factors that are triggered over time: the aging of the immune cells in the skin layers, hormonal changes, and genetic factors, among others [4].

Aging skin is characterized by a reduction in the thickness of the epidermis [5], a flattening of the dermal-epidermal junction, and dermal atrophy owing to the reduction and disorganization of its major extracellular matrix components such as collagen and elastic fibers and of proteoglycans and glycosaminoglycans [6, 7].

Functional alterations noted in the skin of elderly persons include a decreased proliferative potential, loss of responsiveness to growth factors, and a reduction in the production of types I and III collagens with overexpression of extracellular matrix degrading proteases. Eccrine and apocrine secretions are also diminished, and cutaneous immune and inflammatory responses are impaired [8–11].

© Springer International Publishing Switzerland 2016
J.M. Serra-Renom, J.M. Serra-Mestre, *Atlas of Minimally Invasive Facelift*, DOI 10.1007/978-3-319-33018-1_2

2.2 Soft Tissues

2.2.1 Fat Compartments

In recent years, various anatomic [12] and radiologic studies with three-dimensional computed tomographic images [13] have shown that the subcutaneous tissue of the face is divided into different units or compartments that are linked together by connective tissue membranes that stabilize the perforator blood supply to the skin. There are different fat compartments in the superficial planes, located next to the muscles of facial expression, and in the deep planes, found directly on the facial skeleton.

The superficial fat compartments are the nasolabial fat (NLF), superficial medial cheek (SMC), middle cheek, lateral temporal cheek, and the infraorbital fat pad (IOF). Deep compartments constitute the deep medial cheek (DMC) located deep and medial to the NLF and the deep lateral cheek (DLC). The suborbicularis oculi fat (SOOF), which also has a medial and a lateral component, lies deep to the orbicularis oculi muscle of the lower lid. The buccal extension of the buccal fat pad is located just lateral to the DLC.

The deep compartments behave differently from the superficial compartments. Although it is still not known why, the probable differences in fat metabolism and morphology in each of these areas may cause the loss of volume to occur at different rates in different compartments, leading to changes in surface contour [14].

The results of these studies have revolutionized the concept of facial rejuvenation, directing it toward the need not only to correct sagging by techniques that redistribute and reposition tissues but also to provide volume in the areas that are the first to be affected by atrophy in these compartments: the periorbital and malar regions, followed by the lateral cheek, deep cheek, and lateral temporal areas. In fact a topographic map can be generated of the areas that are affected earliest.

2.2.2 Retaining Ligaments

Characterized originally by Furnas [15], the retaining ligaments of the face are osseocutaneous and musculocutaneous fibrous condensations that help to stabilize and support the different structures of the facial region, connecting the dermis and soft tissues to the periosteum of the facial skeleton or the deep muscle fasciae.

Three morphologic types of retaining ligaments have been described. The first are the ones defined as true ligaments: the zygomatic, masseteric, and mandibular ligaments. The second comprise the septae and the superior and inferior temporal facial septae, and the third are the facial adhesions: the temporal adhesion and the lateral orbital thickening (Fig. 2.1) [16].

In fact, the retaining ligaments form the basis for one of the most popular theories of facial aging in recent years—the gravitational theory, based on the fact that the elongation of these ligaments and the loss of their ability to provide support over time generates ptosis in the soft tissues of the face.

2.2.3 Muscle

Although it does not seem that most muscles of facial expression show relevant changes with the passage of time, they do play an important role in other planes such as fat compartments and retaining ligaments through their repeated contraction over the years. In contrast, the skeletal muscles such as the masseter and the temporalis muscles have been reported to atrophy by as much as 50 % [17, 18].

As for the orbicularis oculi and the platysma muscles, which are very thin muscles that cover large areas, the loss of tone in the muscle can generate excess laxity and redundancy.

To date, no studies have specifically analyzed the effects of aging on the facial muscles.

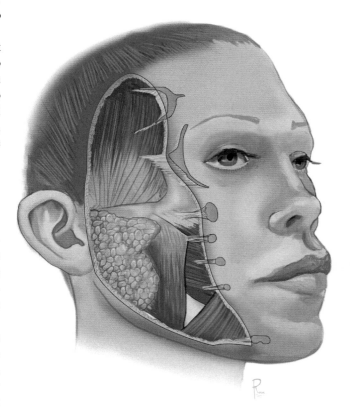

Fig. 2.1 The retaining ligaments of the face (Adapted from Mendelson and Wong [25] with permission)

2.3 The Facial Skeleton

Changes in facial bone structures have a great impact on the aging face. These changes not only involve selective loss of projection in specific areas but also a degree of remodeling resulting from the lack of support of the overlying soft tissue.

The areas most prone to resorption are parts of the orbital rim, the maxilla, the piriform area of the nose, and the prejowl area of the mandible (Fig. 2.2).

2.3.1 The Orbit: Larger Orbital Aperture Area and Width

While the central portions of the upper and lower orbital rims are more stable, the inferolateral part of the orbit is the portion that first shows the tendency to resorb. This tendency can also be observed in the superomedial part of the orbital rim, although at older ages [19, 20].

2.3.2 The Midface: Posterior Displacement and Loss of Projection of the Maxilla and Retrusion of the Piriform Area

The studies by Mendelson and Pessa identified a significant bone resorption with loss of projection of the maxilla, together with a reduction of the jaw angle of about 10° in patients over 60 years. The zygomatic component appears to be more stable than the jaw component in terms of resorption [21–23].

Changes are also observed in the perinasal region. In this area there is an enlargement of the piriform aperture, with a loss of bone, especially in the lower part [22].

2.3.3 Lower Face: Reduced Length and Width of the Jaw and Increase in the Mandibular Angle

Contrary to earlier beliefs, recent research has shown a reduction in the length and height of the jaw, although there are no significant changes in jaw width.

The mandibular angle also increases significantly in both genders with increasing age [24].

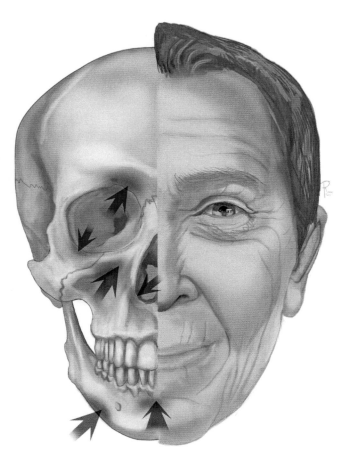

Fig. 2.2 Changes in the facial skeleton with aging. *Arrows* indicate the areas susceptible to resorption with aging (Adapted from Mendelson and Wong [25]; with permission)

References

1. Fisher GJ, Voorhees JJ. Molecular mechanisms of retinoid actions in skin. FASEB J. 1996;10:1002–13.
2. Garmyn M, Yaar M, Boileau N, Backendorf C, Gilchrest BA. Effect of aging and habitual sun exposure on the genetic response of cultured human keratinocytes to solar-simulated irradiation. J Invest Dermatol. 1992;99:743–8.
3. Rexbye H, Petersen I, Johansens M, Klitkou L, Jeune B, Christensen K. Influence of environmental factors on facial ageing. Age Ageing. 2006;35:110–5.
4. Farage MA, Miller KW, Elsner P, Maibach HI. Intrinsic and extrinsic factors in skin ageing: a review. Int J Cosmet Sci. 2008;30:87–95.
5. Lavker RM, Zheng P, Dong G. Aged skin: a study by light, transmission electron, and scanning electron microscopy. J Invest Dermatol. 1987;88:44s–51.
6. Montagna W, Carlisle K. Structural changes in aging human skin. J Invest Dermatol. 1979;73:47–53.
7. Carrino DA, Onnerfjord P, Sandy JD, Cs-Szabo G, Scott PG, Sorrell JM, et al. Age-related changes in the proteoglycans of human skin. Specific cleavage of decorin to yield a major catabolic fragment in adult skin. J Biol Chem. 2003;278:17566–72.
8. Reenstra WR, Yaar M, Gilchrest BA. Effect of donor age on epidermal growth factor processing in man. Exp Cell Res. 1993;209:118–22.
9. Varani J, Dame MK, Rittie L, Cs-Szabo G, Scott PG, Sorrell JM, et al. Decreased collagen production in chronologically aged skin: roles of age-dependent alteration in fibroblast function and defective mechanical stimulation. Am J Pathol. 2006;168:1861–8.
10. West MD, Pereira-Smith OM, Smith JR. Replicative senescence of human skin fibroblasts correlates with a loss of regulation and overexpression of collagenase activity. Exp Cell Res. 1989;184:138–47.
11. Mine S, Fortunel NO, Pageon H, Asselineau D. Aging alters functionally human dermal papillary fibroblasts but not reticular fibroblasts: a new view of skin morphogenesis and aging. PLoS One. 2008;3:e4066.
12. Rohrich RJ, Pessa JE. The fat compartments of the face: anatomy and clinical implications for cosmetic surgery. Plast Reconstr Surg. 2007;119:2219–27; discussion 2228–31.
13. Gierloff M, Stöhring C, Buder T, Wiltfang J. The subcutaneous fat compartments in relation to aesthetically important facial folds and rhytides. J Plast Reconstr Aesthet Surg. 2012;65:1292–7.
14. Wan D, Amirlak B, Giessler P, Rasko Y, Rohrich RJ, Yuan C, Lysikowski J. The differing adipocyte morphologies of deep versus superficial midfacial fat compartments: a cadaveric study. Plast Reconstr Surg. 2014;133:615e–22.
15. Furnas DW. The retaining ligaments of the cheek. Plast Reconstr Surg. 1989;83:11–6.
16. Mendelson BC, Jacobson SR. Surgical anatomy of the midcheek: facial layers, spaces, and the midcheek segments. Clin Plast Surg. 2008;35:395–404.
17. Le Louarn C, Buthiau D, Buis J. Structural aging: the facial recurve concept. Aesthetic Plast Surg. 2007;31:213–8.
18. Le Louarn C. Muscular aging and its involvement in facial aging: the Face Recurve concept. Ann Dermatol Venereol. 2009;136 Suppl 4:S67–72.
19. Pessa JE, Chen Y. Curve analysis of the aging orbital aperture. Plast Reconstr Surg. 2002;109:751–5.
20. Kahn DM, Shaw Jr RB. Aging of the bony orbit: a three-dimensional computed tomographic study. Aesthet Surg J. 2008;28:258–64.
21. Pessa JE. An algorithm of facial aging: verification of Lambros's theory by three-dimensional stereolithography, with reference to the pathogenesis of midfacial aging, scleral show, and the lateral suborbital trough deformity. Plast Reconstr Surg. 2000;106:479–88.
22. Shaw Jr RB, Kahn DM. Aging of the midface bony elements: a three-dimensional computed tomographic study. Plast Reconstr Surg. 2007;119:675–81.
23. Mendelson BC, Hartley W, Scott M, McNab A, Granzow JW. Age-related changes of the orbit and midcheek and the implications for facial rejuvenation. Aesthetic Plast Surg. 2007;31:419–23.
24. Shaw Jr RB, Katzel EB, Koltz PF, Kahn DM, Girotto JA, Langstein HN. Aging of the mandible and its aesthetic implications. Plast Reconstr Surg. 2010;125:33.
25. Mendelson B, Wong CH. Anatomy of the aging face. In: Neligan PC, editor. Plastic surgery. 3rd ed. London: Elsevier; 2013. p. 78–92.

Fat Grafting: Principles and General Concepts

Soft tissue defects and asymmetries represent a common challenge for surgeons in their clinical practice. To correct these problems, surgical techniques are applied in order to obtain healthy tissue from other body regions. Alternatively, a variety of filling materials are available for use; however, although good short-term results are achieved with the vast majority of fillers, some of them are associated with significant complications such as extrusion or migration of the injected material, hypersensitivity reactions, and infections [1, 2].

The idea of attempting to reconstruct a defect with the same or similar material following one of the Converse principles has led many surgeons to test the use of autologous fat grafts as fillers. The evolution of these grafts has changed since the advent of liposuction and the later standardization of atraumatic structural fat grafting in the late 1990s (Fig. 3.1) [3].

Since the standardization of the technique described by Coleman [4, 5], a great many clinical applications have been reported to increase volume and to improve the quality of the tissue [6], as in the case of irradiated tissues after oncology surgery for the breast [7] or the head and neck [8]. However, fat is also frequently studied in the field of tissue engineering as a rich source of cells with regenerative capacity [9].

Fat offers many advantages as a filler. It is an autologous material that is nontoxic, biocompatible, nonimmunogenic, and nonirritant, and it does not migrate. It possesses similar physical features to the tissue in which it is to be implanted, and its procurement is straightforward using low-pressure liposuction. It is also relatively inexpensive. Another advantage to consider when using it as a filler is its inherent capacity to improve the quality of the tissues and the skin, rejuvenating the area into which it has been injected.

Approximately 30 % of aspirated fat cells are mature adipocytes. The remaining two-thirds are formed by a very diverse cell population, also known as the stromal vascular fraction (SVF), which mainly comprises fibroblasts, connective tissue fibers, endothelial cells and their progenitors, immunomodulatory cells (e.g., macrophages, lymphocytes), and adipose-derived stem cells (ADSCs) [10].

However, the disadvantage of fat is that it is a partially absorbable material. As a graft that obtains nutrients through plasmatic diffusion from the start of the procedure until vascularization is restored, some of its cells will undergo apoptosis. This issue has been studied in depth by Eto et al. [11] and by Kato et al. [12]. These authors described three zones in each of the "cylinder" of fat injected: the outermost part, which is in direct contact with the receiving area and is called the surviving zone; an intermediate area called the regenerating zone; and the innermost part called the necrotic zone.

In the surviving zone, both adipocytes and ADSCs survive. In the regenerating zone, the adipocytes undergo apoptosis, but the ADSCs survive because they are more resistant to situations of hypoxia. The adipocyte apoptosis generates a series of signals to the ADSCs to initiate differentiation and proliferation processes to become preadipocytes and later mature adipocytes. However, in the necrotic zone, both adipocytes and ADSCs die; there is no cell replacement, and scar tissue cysts or oily cysts are formed.

Precisely in order to increase the retention of the injected volume and the survival of the fat, many surgeons have tried to enrich the fat with SVF cells [13] or by using other prosurvival strategies such as platelet-rich plasma (PRP) [14], improving the conditions in the receiving area [15] or studying each of the stages of its preparation.

With the increasing amount of experimental and clinical data available regarding the technical aspects, we will

© Springer International Publishing Switzerland 2016
J.M. Serra-Renom, J.M. Serra-Mestre, *Atlas of Minimally Invasive Facelift*, DOI 10.1007/978-3-319-33018-1_3

Fig. 3.1 Historical overview of autologous fat injection

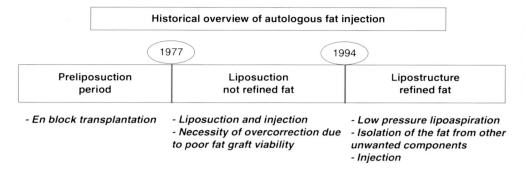

briefly review the preparation of the fat from its harvesting to its injection.

3.1 Fat Harvesting

3.1.1 Donor Site Selection

According to the Current Literature [16–22]
- There are no significant differences in fat graft retention volume between abdominal and nonabdominal areas. However, the lower abdomen and inner thighs may have a higher adipose-derived stem cells concentration than other areas.
- The choice of the donor site depends on the ease and safety of access, the patient's preferences, and the amount of fat available.

Ease and safety of access are not the only criteria to bear in mind in the choice of the donor site: the enhancement of the patient's contour should also be considered. When deciding to obtain fat from an area of the lower limbs or the flanks, the need for liposuction of the contralateral side should also be assessed.

Incisions should be placed whenever possible in previous scars or natural skin folds or otherwise in areas that are covered by clothing (preferably those covered by underwear).

In general—and especially when harvesting fat for the facial region given the smaller volumes of fat required—we try to use areas in which any small irregularity or sequel after liposuction is not noticeable to the patient. The insides of the knees and the thighs are good examples; in contrast, irregularities in the abdomen are highly visible. The internal sides of the knees and thighs are locations where thin or athletic young women tend to have higher amounts of fat.

3.1.2 Tumescent Solution

According to the Current Literature [23–28]
- A tumescent solution is a dilution of a local anesthetic (LA) and a vasoconstrictor in a large volume of fluid. It reduces pain and bleeding and facilitates liposuction.
- Some studies suggest that LA may modulate isolated preadipocyte viability rates. However, at the doses used and with brief exposure of the fat to anesthetic agents, there does not seem to be a detrimental effect on the grafts.
- Furthermore no significant differences have been observed between the commonly used anesthetic drugs, with the exception of articaine delivered with epinephrine.
- The LA most frequently used for liposuction and fat grafting is lidocaine. Klein proposed a safe limit dose in a tumescent solution of 30–35 mL/kg. Other studies suggested that doses up to 55 mL/kg can be used with minimal risk of lidocaine toxicity.

Fat grafting can be performed under general, epidural, or local anesthesia with or without sedation.

When surgery is performed under local anesthesia, 2 h prior to surgery the extraction area (previously indicated to the patient during a presurgery visit) is covered with a topical anesthetic cream. The tumescent solution contains 0.05 % lidocaine in a saline solution and 1:200,000 epinephrine.

When the procedure is performed under general anesthetic, the tumescence can be done with a vasoconstrictor alone diluted in saline solution or by adding low concentrations of local anesthetic (the authors' preference is 0.02 % lidocaine).

Infiltration should be performed slowly, avoiding sudden movements to ensure maximum patient comfort, especially when general anesthesia and sedation are not used. In general, the infiltrated volume is usually about the same as the volume of aspirated fat (1:1 ratio).

After waiting about 20 min for the tumescence to take effect, the liposuction is initiated.

3.1.3 Selection of the Harvesting Cannula

According to the Current Literature [29–34]
- Reports comparing multiperforated cannulas with the Coleman 3-mm aspiration cannula have shown no significant difference in cell viability or size of the engrafted fat tissue.
- Experimental studies comparing the diameter of the cannula found that a larger diameter enhances cell viability. However, most of these studies used a dry technique with a nontumescent solution.

Multiple cannulas are available with a variety of diameters with one or more orifices through which the fat is aspirated and with orifices with blunt or cutting surfaces. In general, they all have a blunt tip in order to keep trauma to a minimum.

To obtain structural fat grafting or macrofat, a 3-mm cannula is normally used. If the aim is to obtain microfat grafts, whether they are to be injected via a cannula or a needle (in the case of sharp-needle intradermal fat grafting (SNIF)), 2.4-mm microport harvester cannulas with barbed and beveled 1-mm ports are very useful. Currently, two commercial firms manufacture them: Tulip Medical Products (San Diego, CA) and Wells Johnson (Tucson, AZ).

3.1.4 Liposuction

According to the Current Literature [35–44]
- The methods used to harvest fat are handheld syringe aspiration and vacuum-assisted, water-assisted, or ultrasound-assisted lipectomy.
- Current evidence does not support one harvesting technique over the others, even though some studies indicate differences in cell viability and adipocyte functionality with the use of these different isolation methods.
- Techniques that use low-pressure suction appear to improve adipocyte viability and have less fibrosis.

In our everyday practice, when small amounts of fat are required, we use handheld syringe aspiration connected to a 10-mL syringe with a Luer-lock tip. This results in a suction pressure of about 0.37 atm. If larger quantities of fat are required, we perform suction-assisted lipectomy, with the liposuction device at a low pressure (0.5 atm).

To avoid irregularities in the liposuctioned area and to obtain the best possible result in the donor area, the following points should be borne in mind:

1. During liposuction, it is advisable to change the site and the direction of the aspirations and to crisscross the tunnels from two different incisions whenever possible.
2. After liposuction, and once the fat extraction is completed, the donor site should be regularized using a flat liposuction cannula without aspiration prior to suturing the incisions with a 5-0 monofilament suture.

3.2 Fat Processing Techniques

According to the Current Literature [45–60]
- The processing techniques for fat grafts are centrifugation, filtration, washing, and Telfa rolling.
- When all the data are evaluated, no one technique emerges as clearly superior to the others. There is still a high degree of discordance because of the inconsistent results from animal and human studies.
- When centrifugation is used, several studies note that forces greater than 3000 rpm (1200 g) cause more cell damage. To establish the amount of "g" to be applied, the radius of the rotor of the centrifuge must be known.

Processing techniques are intended to isolate the adipose tissue aspirated from the oil, blood, and debris and other unwanted components of the tumescence solution. This is important because these elements may adversely affect the viability and retention of the fat graft. To isolate the fat, the following techniques are available:

3.2.1 Centrifugation

There is a disagreement regarding the rpm and time that the fat should be centrifuged. Coleman [4, 5] reported 3000 rpm for 3 min, while we use 2000 rpm for 2 min.

After centrifugation, three levels can be observed in the syringe. The lower one contains blood and debris, water, and components of the tumescence solution; the middle layer consists of the fat to be injected; and the top layer is formed by the oil resulting from the broken down fatty acids.

To separate the hematic level, the bottom plug is opened, and the blood is allowed to flow out onto a tray. The broken down fatty acids in the top level can be removed by decantation, and if necessary the oil can be removed with the aid of a small lined gauze. Currently closed methods are available for separating these undesired components after centrifugation.

3.2.2   Washing and Filtration

In this process, the fat is separated from the other components to be used by washing and filtering with saline solution. Both closed and open filter units are reported.

3.2.3   Washing and Decantation

For washing and decantation, we favor the use of a closed circuit. We aspirate 5 mL of fat with the syringe and then fill the other half with 4 mL of saline solution. After decanting the fat and removing the supernatant, we repeat the maneuver until the fat is clean.

3.2.4   Telfa Rolling

This procedure consists of pouring the aspirated fat onto large pieces of Telfa nonadherent dressings. The fat is gently rolled and kneaded around the gauze and then transferred back again into the syringes.

Once the fat has been obtained, it is passed into 1 mL syringes via a Luer-lock transfer connector.

3.3   Fat Injection

According to the Current Literature [33, 61–64]
- Injections may be done in multiple passes, in multiple tissue planes, and in multiple directions, injecting small volumes in each pass.
- At present, overcorrection to obtain better graft survival seems to lack scientific support.
- Compressive bandages or massages on the grafted area should be avoided.

Some authors consider the moment of injection as the most important part of the process.

In general, and when there is no fibrosis, the fat should be injected with blunt cannulas. However, when there are scar retractions or fibrosis, sharp needles can be used to release them before injection of the fat in order to avoid damaging nerves, vessels, or other anatomic structures. In cases in which fat needs to be injected into more superficial subdermal planes, direct injection with a needle can also be useful.

These grafts should deposit small amounts of fat in each pass, thereby enhancing graft survival and the integration of the adipose tissue implanted into the recipient site.

First we introduce the cannula without infiltrating and then infiltrate as we withdraw it. This creates an effect like beads on a necklace, generating several levels of injection, and the procedure must be repeated several times at different levels. It is also very important to introduce the fat into different areas to create a mesh or crisscross pattern and to make tunnels at all levels so as to prevent the accumulation of fat.

References

1. Rzany B, DeLorenzi C. Understanding, avoiding, and managing severe filler complications. Plast Reconstr Surg. 2015;136(5 Suppl): 196S–203.
2. Sorensen EP, Urman C. Cosmetic complications: rare and serious events following botulinum toxin and soft tissue filler administration. J Drugs Dermatol. 2015;14:486–91.
3. Mojallal A, Foyatier JL. Historique de l'utilisation du tissu adipeux comme produit de comblement en chirurgie plastique. Ann Chir Plast Esthet. 2004;49:419–25.
4. Coleman SR. Lipoinfiltration in the upper lip white roll. Aesth Surg. 1994;14:231–4.
5. Coleman SR. Long term survival of fat transplants: controlled demonstrations. Aesthetic Plast Surg. 1995;19:421–5.
6. Mazzola RF, Mazzola IC. History of fat grafting: from ram fat to stem cells. Clin Plast Surg. 2015;42:147–53.
7. Serra-Renom JM, Muñoz-Olmo JL, Serra-Mestre JM. Fat grafting in postmastectomy breast reconstruction with expanders and prostheses in patients who have received radiotherapy: formation of new subcutaneous tissue. Plast Reconstr Surg. 2010;125:12–8.
8. Karmali RJ, Nguyen AT, Skoracki RJ, et al. Outcomes following autologous fat grafting in head and neck oncologic reconstruction. Plast Reconstr Surg. 2015;136(4 Suppl):49–50.
9. Laschke MW, Menger MD. Adipose tissue-derived microvascular fragments: natural vascularization units for regenerative medicine. Trends Biotechnol. 2015;33:442–8.
10. Avram AS, Avram MM, James WD. Subcutaneous fat in normal and diseased states: 2. Anatomy and physiology of white and brown adipose tissue. J Am Acad Dermatol. 2005;53:671–83.
11. Eto H, Kato H, Suga H, Aoi N, Doi K, Kuno S, Yoshimura K. The fate of adipocytes after nonvascularized fat grafting: evidence of early death and replacement of adipocytes. Plast Reconstr Surg. 2012;129:1081–92.
12. Kato H, Mineda K, Eto H, Doi K, Kuno S, Kinoshita K, et al. Degeneration, regeneration, and cicatrization after fat grafting: dynamic total tissue remodeling during the first 3 months. Plast Reconstr Surg. 2014;133:303e–13.

13. Kakudo N, Tanaka Y, Morimoto N, Ogawa T, Kushida S, Hara T, Kusumoto K. Adipose-derived regenerative cell (ADRC)-enriched fat grafting: optimal cell concentration and effects on grafted fat characteristics. J Transl Med. 2013;11:254.

14. Serra-Mestre JM, Serra-Renom JM, Martinez L, Almadori A, D'Andrea F. Platelet-rich plasma mixed-fat grafting: a reasonable prosurvival strategy for fat grafts? Aesthetic Plast Surg. 2014;38:1041–9.

15. Forbes SJ, Rosenthal N. Preparing the ground for tissue regeneration: from mechanism to therapy. Nat Med. 2014;20:857–69.

16. Rohrich RJ, Sorokin ES, Brown SA. In search of improved fat transfer viability: a quantitative analysis of the role of centrifugation and harvest site. Plast Reconstr Surg. 2004;113:391–5.

17. Ullmann Y, Shoshani O, Fodor A, Ramon Y, Carmi N, Eldor L, Gilhar A. Searching for the favorable donor site for fat injection: in vivo study using the nude mice model. Dermatol Surg. 2005;31:1304–7.

18. Padoin AV, Braga-Silva J, Martins P, Rezende K, Rezende AR, Grechi B, et al. Sources of processed lipoaspirate cells: influence of donor site on cell concentration. Plast Reconstr Surg. 2008;122:614–8.

19. Kishi K, Imanishi N, Ohara H, Ninomiya R, Okabe K, Hattori N, et al. Distribution of adipose-derived stem cells in adipose tissues from human cadavers. J Plast Reconstr Aesthet Surg. 2010;63:1717.

20. Lim AA, Fan K, Allam KA, Wan D, Tabit C, Liao E, et al. Autologous fat transplantation in the craniofacial patient. J Craniofac Surg. 2012;23:1061–6.

21. Li K, Gao J, Zhang Z, Li J, Cha P, Liao Y, et al. Selection of donor site for fat grafting and cell isolation. Aesthetic Plast Surg. 2013;37:153–8.

22. Small K, Choi M, Petruolo O, Lee C, Karp N. Is there an ideal donor site of fat for secondary breast reconstruction? Aesthet Surg J. 2014;34:545–50.

23. Moore Jr JH, Kolaczynski JW, Morales LM, Considine RV, Pietrzkowski Z, Noto PF, Caro JF. Viability of fat obtained by syringe suction lipectomy: effects of local anesthesia with lidocaine. Aesthetic Plast Surg. 1995;19:335–9.

24. Kim IH, Yang JD, Lee DG, Chung HY, Cho BC. Evaluation of centrifugation technique and effect of epinephrine on fat cell viability in autologous fat injection. Aesthet Surg J. 2009;29:35–9.

25. Shoshani O, Berger J, Fodor L, Ramon Y, Shupak A, Kehat I, et al. The effect of lidocaine and adrenaline on the viability of injected adipose tissue: an experimental study in nude mice. J Drugs Dermatol. 2005;4:311–6.

26. Keck M, Zeyda M, Gollinger K, Burjak S, Kamolz LP, Frey M, Stulnig TM. Local anesthetics have a major impact on viability of preadipocytes and their differentiation into adipocytes. Plast Reconstr Surg. 2010;126:1500–5.

27. Livaoğlu M, Buruk CK, Uraloğlu M, Ersöz S, Livaoğlu A, Sözen E, Agdoğan Ö. Effects of lidocaine plus epinephrine and prilocaine on autologous fat graft survival. J Craniofac Surg. 2012;23:1015–8.

28. Agostini T, Lazzeri D, Pini A, Marino G, Li Quattrini A, Bani D, Dini M. Wet and dry techniques for structural fat graft harvesting. Plast Reconstr Surg. 2012;130:331e–9.

29. Shiffman MA, Mirrafati S. Fat transfer techniques: the effect of harvest and transfer methods on adipocyte viability and review of the literature. Dermatol Surg. 2001;27:819–26.

30. Özsoy Z, Kul Z, Bilir A. The role of cannula diameter in improved adipocyte viability: a quantitative analysis. Aesthet Surg J. 2006;26:287–9.

31. Erdim M, Tezel E, Numanoglu A, Sav A. The effects of the size of liposuction cannula on adipocyte survival and the optimum temperature for fat graft storage: an experimental study. J Plast Reconstr Aesthet Surg. 2009;62:1210–4.

32. Kirkham JC, Lee JH, Medina MA, McCormack MC, Randolph MA, Austen Jr WG. The impact of liposuction cannula size on adipocyte viability. Ann Plast Surg. 2012;69:479–81.

33. Nguyen PS, Desouches C, Gay AM, Hautier A, Magalon G. Development of micro-injection as an innovative autologous fat graft technique: the use of adipose tissue as dermal filler. J Plast Reconstr Aesthet Surg. 2012;65:1692–9.

34. Alharbi Z, Opländer C, Almakadi S, Fritz A, Vogt M, Pallua N. Conventional vs. micro-fat harvesting: how fat harvesting technique affects tissue-engineering approaches using adipose tissue-derived stem/stromal cells. J Plast Reconstr Aesthet Surg. 2013;66:1271–8.

35. Rohrich RJ, Morales DE, Krueger JE, Ansari M, Ochoa O, Robinson Jr J, Beran SJ. Comparative lipoplasty analysis of in vivo-treated adipose tissue. Plast Reconstr Surg. 2000;105:2152–8.

36. Pu LL, Cui X, Fink BF, Cibull ML, Gao D. The viability of fatty tissue within adipose aspirates after conventional liposuction: a comprehensive study. Ann Plast Surg. 2005;54:288–92.

37. Smith P, Adams Jr WP, Lipschitz AH, Chau B, Sorokin E, Rohrich RJ, Brown SA. Autologous human fat grafting: effect of harvesting and preparation techniques on adipocyte graft survival. Plast Reconstr Surg. 2006;117:1836–44.

38. Pu LL, Coleman SR, Cui X, Ferguson Jr RE, Vasconez HC. Autologous fat grafts harvested and refined by the Coleman technique: a comparative study. Plast Reconstr Surg. 2008;122:932–7.

39. Crawford JL, Hubbard BA, Colbert SH, Puckett CL. Fine tuning lipoaspirate viability for fat grafting. Plast Reconstr Surg. 2010;126:1342–8.

40. Lee JH, Kirkham JC, McCormack MC, Nicholls AM, Randolph MA, Austen Jr WG. The effect of pressure and shear on autologous fat grafting. Plast Reconstr Surg. 2013;131:1125–36.

41. Fisher C, Grahovac TL, Schafer ME, Shippert RD, Marra KG, Rubin JP. Comparison of harvest and processing techniques for fat grafting and adipose stem cell isolation. Plast Reconstr Surg. 2013;132:351–61.

42. Schafer ME, Hicok KC, Mills DC, Cohen SR, Chao JJ. Acute adipocyte viability after third-generation ultrasound-assisted liposuction. Aesthet Surg J. 2013;33:698–704.

43. Keck M, Kober J, Riedl O, Kitzinger HB, Wolf S, Stulnig TM, et al. Power assisted liposuction to obtain adipose-derived stem cells: impact on viability and differentiation to adipocytes in comparison to manual aspiration. J Plast Reconstr Aesthet Surg. 2014;67:e1–8.

44. Yin S, Luan J, Fu S, Wang Q, Zhuang Q. Does water-jet force make a difference in fat grafting? In vitro and in vivo evidence of improved lipoaspirate viability and fat graft survival. Plast Reconstr Surg. 2015;135:127–38.

45. Boschert MT, Beckert BW, Puckett CL, Concannon MJ. Analysis of lipocyte viability after liposuction. Plast Reconstr Surg. 2002;109:761–5; discussion 766–7.

46. Butterwick KJ. Lipoaugmentation for aging hands: a comparison of the longevity and aesthetic results of centrifuged versus noncentrifuged fat. Dermatol Surg. 2002;28:987–91.

47. Ramon Y, Shoshani O, Peled IJ, Gilhar A, Carmi N, Fodor L. Enhancing the take of injected adipose tissue by a simple method for concentrating fat cells. Plast Reconstr Surg. 2005;115:197–201.

48. Rose JG, Lucarelli MJ, Lemke BN, Dortzbach RK, Boxrud CA, Obagi S, Patel S. Histologic comparison of autologous fat processing methods. Ophthal Plast Reconstr Surg. 2006;22:195–200.

49. Kurita M, Matsumoto D, Shigeura T, Sato K, Gonda K, Harii K, et al. Influences of centrifugation on cells and tissues in liposuction aspirates: optimized centrifugation for lipotransfer and cell isolation. Plast Reconstr Surg. 2008;121:1033–41.

50. Khater R, Atanassova P, Anastassov Y, Pellerin P, Martinot-Duquennoy V. Clinical and experimental study of autologous fat grafting after processing by centrifugation and serum lavage. Aesthetic Plast Surg. 2009;33:37–43.

51. Condé-Green A, de Amorim NF, Pitanguy I. Influence of decantation, washing and centrifugation on adipocyte and mesenchymal

stem cell content of aspirated adipose tissue: a comparative study. J Plast Reconstr Aesthet Surg. 2010;63:1375–81.

52. Condé-Green A, Baptista LS, de Amorin NF, de Oliveira ED, da Silva KR, Pedrosa Cda S. Effects of centrifugation on cell composition and viability of aspirated adipose tissue processed for transplantation. Aesthet Surg J. 2010;30:249–55.

53. Xie Y, Zheng D, Li Q, Chen Y, Lei H, Pu LL. The effect of centrifugation on viability of fat grafts: an evaluation with the glucose transport test. J Plast Reconstr Aesthet Surg. 2010;63:482–7.

54. Zhu M, Zhou Z, Chen Y, Schreiber R, Ransom JT, Fraser JK, et al. Supplementation of fat grafts with adipose-derived regenerative cells improves long-term graft retention. Ann Plast Surg. 2010;64:222–8.

55. Minn KW, Min KH, Chang H, Kim S, Heo EJ. Effects of fat preparation methods on the viabilities of autologous fat grafts. Aesthetic Plast Surg. 2010;34:626–31.

56. Botti G, Pascali M, Botti C, Bodog F, Cervelli V. A clinical trial in facial fat grafting: filtered and washed versus centrifuged fat. Plast Reconstr Surg. 2011;127:2464–73.

57. Ferraro GA, De Francesco F, Tirino V, Cataldo C, Rossano F, Nicoletti G, D'Andrea F. Effects of a new centrifugation method on adipose cell viability for autologous fat grafting. Aesthetic Plast Surg. 2011;35:341–8.

58. Pulsfort AK, Wolter TP, Pallua N. The effect of centrifugal forces on viability of adipocytes in centrifuged lipoaspirates. Ann Plast Surg. 2011;66:292–5.

59. Hoareau L, Bencharif K, Girard AC, Delarue P, Hulard O, Festy F, et al. Effect of centrifugation and washing on adipose graft viability: a new method to improve graft efficiency. J Plast Reconstr Aesthet Surg. 2013;66:712–9.

60. Pfaff M, Wu W, Zellner E, Steinbacher DM. Processing technique for lipofilling influences adipose-derived stem cell concentration and cell viability in lipoaspirate. Aesthetic Plast Surg. 2014;38:224–9.

61. Dasiou-Plakida D. Fat injections for facial rejuvenation: 17 years experience in 1720 patients. J Cosmet Dermatol. 2003;2:119–25.

62. Trepsat F. Midface reshaping with micro-fat grafting. Ann Chir Plast Esthet. 2009;54:435–43.

63. Mazzola RF. Fat injection: from filling to regeneration. St. Louis: Quality Medical Publishing; 2009. p. 373–422.

64. Tonnard P, Verpaele A, Peeters G, Hamdi M, Cornelissen M, Declercq H. Nanofat grafting: basic research and clinical applications. Plast Reconstr Surg. 2013;132:1017–26.

Anatomic Reference Points to Consider to Avoid Vessel and Nerve Injury During Facial Fat Grafting

4

Before performing fat grafting, it is important to consider the possible risk areas [1, 2]. It is very useful to mark reference points for identifying areas where vessels and nerves are likely to be near the surface. This is done with an easily washable pen because vigorous washing at the end of the procedure would increase the risk of mobilizing the fat graft.

Damage to blood vessels or obstruction is rare, especially when cannulas are used. However, the recent increase in the use of sharp needles or thin cannulas below 1 mm in diameter raises the risk of complications. Complications are also possible in cases requiring the release of scar adhesions in previously operated or radiated areas. In general, blunt cannulas should always be used when fat grafting is performed in deep planes; needle injection should be limited to very superficial intradermal or subdermal planes.

Another important point is that aspiration should be performed prior to fat injection to ensure that no vessels have been punctured. Retrograde injection is performed, injecting small amounts of fat as the cannula is withdrawn. Injections with short, quick in and out movements have become popular, but in our view, they may cause lesions in the small nerve branches of the facial and trigeminal nerves. The introduction of the cannula in facial fat grafting should be slow, without forcing, and once introduced, the cannula or needle should be gradually withdrawn and small amounts of fat introduced continuously, avoiding the formation of deposits.

4.1 Medial Forehead and Glabella

The two important components of this area are the supraorbital and supratrochlear neurovascular bundle, branches of the trigeminal nerve, and the ophthalmic artery. They are easy to identify if the midpupillary line is taken as a reference point.

4.1.1 Supraorbital Neurovascular Bundle

To identify the exit point of the supraorbital nerve and vessels, the midpupillary line can be used, drawing a straight line from the pupil at its intersection with the eyebrow line. This point, which corresponds to the supraorbital notch, is located around 2.7 cm from the midline [1].

The nerve passes cranially toward the front muscle below the corrugator muscle. The supraorbital vessels divide into superficial and deep branches, anastomosing medially with the supratrochlear artery and laterally with the superficial temporal artery.

When the tail of the eyebrow is raised, fat is injected in a subcutaneous plane. It is important not to reach the supraorbital bundle because this would cause injury.

4.1.2 Supratrochlear Neurovascular Bundle

Approximately 1 cm medial to the supraorbital nerve exit point, the supratrochlear nerve and vessels are identified. From its exit, the nerve passes cranially and enters the corrugator muscle, dividing into several branches. The artery runs cranially, anastomosing with both the supraorbital artery and the supratrochlear artery of the opposite side [1].

4.2 Temple and Lateral Forehead

4.2.1 Superficial Temporal Vessels and Their Branches

The artery, a branch of the external carotid artery, is easily palpable in the preauricular region approximately 1 cm above and below the tragus. Once past the zygomatic process, it runs upward within the temporal fascia surface and then divides into the frontal and parietal branches [1, 2].

© Springer International Publishing Switzerland 2016
J.M. Serra-Renom, J.M. Serra-Mestre, *Atlas of Minimally Invasive Facelift*, DOI 10.1007/978-3-319-33018-1_4

In this area it is important to remember the superficial temporal venous plexus, and so it is advisable to use a cannula for the injection.

4.2.2 Temporal Branch of the Facial Nerve

Schematically, we can draw a triangle where the nerve lies on the undersurface of the temporoparietal fascia. This triangle runs from 0.5 cm below the tragus to 2 cm above the lateral eyebrow and from this point to the lateral canthus [1]. Injury will affect the frontal muscle, creating a brow ptosis and asymmetry with respect to the contralateral side.

4.3 Cheek and Nasal Area

4.3.1 Facial Angular Artery (from the Oral Commissure)

This artery follows a winding route from the oral commissure to the nasal ala along the nasolabial folds. It is identified approximately 1.5–2 cm lateral to the oral commissure and around 0.6–1 cm lateral to the nasal ala. Along its route it passes at a depth of 1 cm, although this is variable. From the nasal ala, it runs cranially to the nasopalpebral angle, where the angular artery anastomoses with the nasal artery, which is a branch of the ophthalmic artery [1, 2].

4.3.2 Infraorbital Neurovascular Bundle

Its exit point is approximately 1–1.5 cm from the inferior orbital rim, directly below the midpupillary line [1].

The artery contributes mainly to the irrigation of the lower eyelid, lacrimal sac, upper lip, and the lateral aspect of the nose. It anastomoses with the transverse facial artery, the buccal artery, and branches of the facial and ophthalmic arteries. The infraorbital nerve innervates the lower eyelid, the upper lip, and part of the nasal vestibule.

This area should be paid particular attention to when fat grafting of the malar region is performed and when cannulas are used.

4.3.3 Dorsal Nasal Artery

This artery exits via the superomedial apex of the orbit, passing above the medial palpebral ligament and then anastomoses with the angular artery [2]. Although the nasal dorsum has a good blood supply, its vessels are very small; therefore, the potential risk of complications caused by the injection of fillers or fat is very small or nonexistent.

4.3.4 Transverse Facial Artery

This artery originates at the level of the mandibular condyle from the superficial temporal artery and passes below the zygomatic arch until reaching the cheek [2].

4.3.5 Buccal Branch of the Facial Artery

From its origin in the maxillary artery between the insertion of the temporal muscle and the medial pterygoid, the buccal branch runs obliquely and surfaces toward the buccinator muscle. It undergoes various anastomoses with branches of the facial and infraorbital arteries [2].

4.3.6 Zygomatic and Buccal Branches of the Facial Nerve

These nerves can be identified by drawing a triangle whose vertices are the mandibular angle, the oral commissure, and the point of maximum projection of the malar eminence [2]. This is the area of activity of these two branches of the facial nerve that are responsible for the mobility of the upper lip and mouth.

4.4 Perioral Area and Lower Third of the Face

4.4.1 Facial Artery (Toward the Oral Commissure)

This artery is related to the lower edge of the jaw and later to the anterior edge of the masseter muscle, from where it continues to the oral commissure. It is covered by the platysma muscle and the depressor muscle of the angle of the mouth [2].

4.4.2 Superior and Inferior Labial Arteries

These are branches of the facial artery that originate at the level of the oral commissure and pass toward the midline, where they anastomose with the labial arteries of the opposite side. They are located behind the muscular plane [2].

4.4.3 Marginal Mandibular Branch

This branch can be identified in the mandible approximately 2 cm lateral to the oral commissure. At this point, by drawing a circle of around 2 cm, we can define the area where the nerve surfaces [2].

Injury to this branch creates an asymmetry in the mouth, which is most evident while smiling. The function of the branch is to mobilize the depressor muscles of the lower lip and the corner of the mouth.

4.4.4 Mental Nerve

In the middle of the jaw, below the second premolar, is the mental nerve, which is responsible for the sensitivity of half of the lower lip [2].

4.5 Cervical Area

For the treatment of cervical horizontal wrinkles, it is very important to perform the injection in a very superficial plane. In the subdermal space, a cannula is always used; then the needle is used in an intradermal plane following the lines of the wrinkle. In this area, extreme care must be taken with the external jugular veins and the anterior cervical vessels.

References

1. Seckel BR. Facial danger zones: avoiding nerve injury in facial plastic surgery. 2nd ed. St. Louis: Quality Medical Publishing Inc; 2010.
2. Pessa JE, Rohrich RJ. Facial topography: clinical anatomy of the face. St. Louis: Quality Medical Publishing Inc; 2012.

The injection of fat in the facial region is a relatively safe procedure. When performed correctly, the complication rate is low [1, 2].

Although most complications described after fat injection in the facial region refer to aesthetic aspects such as irregularities or asymmetries, several serious complications have been reported. Evidently, surgeons need to be aware of these situations in order to prevent them.

Currently, the development of new forms of injection with small diameter cannulas or sharp needles has improved the results and made it possible to correct areas where until recently fat grafting could not be performed. Examples are in the eyelids and the tear trough, where the skin is very thin. In these areas in particular, great care is needed with regard to the selection of the correct volume of fat to be injected and the depth of injection, especially when using sharp needles, in order to prevent damage to vessels or other structures. When needles are used instead of cannulas, the injection should be dermal or subdermal; injections in the deep subcutaneous plane should be avoided.

The main complications to consider when performing facial fat grafting follow.

5.1 Bruising and Swelling

A certain degree of surface bruising and swelling is normal during the first 2 weeks after surgery. It is important to inform the patient of this, especially in the case of nanofat grafting in the periorbital region, when the bruising usually lasts longer—up to 4 or 5 weeks [3].

Chronic inflammation or swelling in the eyelid has very occasionally been reported in the literature [4]. In these cases, reoperation may be required to extract fat.

5.2 Infection

As with all surgical procedures, it is essential to prevent bacterial contamination of the graft. This is done by using a sterile technique and the preoperative preparation of the donor and recipient areas.

There do not appear to be any great differences between the uses of open or closed methods for the processing of the fat graft when it is performed in the operating room using a sterile technique [1].

5.3 Accumulations or Cysts

Distributing the fat in multiple planes during the injection and taking care not to inject all the fat in one place avoid irregularities and the formation of oil cysts in the injected area. In the area of the eyelids and tear trough, where the dermal component is practically nonexistent, the formation of irregularities visible to the naked eye is common if fine microfat grafting cannulas are not used.

In this area especially, great care must be taken to inject only a small amount of fat and also to place it below the orbicularis muscle.

If irregularities appear after the injection of fat, the area should be massaged until they disappear.

5.4 Asymmetries

Prior to surgery, the vast majority of patients present small asymmetries between the two sides of the face. The surgeon must identify them during the preoperative evaluation and mention their existence to the patient.

J.M. Serra-Renom, J.M. Serra-Mestre, *Atlas of Minimally Invasive Facelift*, DOI 10.1007/978-3-319-33018-1_5

During the intraoperative phase, it helps to divide the face into different compartments or areas and to count the amount of fat that is injected into each of the areas on both sides. The symmetry should also be assessed as the fat is injected.

5.5 Reabsorption

Inevitably, some of the fat is reabsorbed. Although we believe that the degree of reabsorption depends on the technique and also the surgeon's experience, changes in the weight of the patient may play an important role. In reviewing the literature, whether or not prosurvival strategies such as the fat-enriched stromal vascular fraction, platelet-rich plasma, or second-generation platelet-rich fibrin (PRP) are used [5], reabsorption of around 40–50 % of the injected volume has been reported [6–8].

5.6 Hypo- or Hypercorrection

In this connection, the surgeon's experience with the technique is particularly relevant. In our opinion, especially early in the surgeon's career, hypocorrection is preferable because there will always be time to carry out any necessary retouches.

5.7 Fat Embolism

Although it is a rare complication, some cases of blindness have been reported [9–13], probably related to retinal ischemia caused by embolization of the ophthalmic and central arteries and also to occasional cases of cerebral infarction after facial fat grafting [9, 10]. To avoid this complication, it is important to use blunt cannulas, to inject the fat while withdrawing, and always to aspirate before injecting. When sharp needles are used, the injection must always be superficial. In our opinion, although needle techniques are useful in some cases, they should never be used in deep planes, and great care must be taken when injecting into the periorbital and glabellar regions and the nasolabial fold so as not to damage the angular artery.

5.8 Damage to Anatomic Structures (Nerves, Arteries, Muscle, Parotid, or Other Glands)

Complications can occur, especially in cases of reconstructive surgery in which fibrous attachments are released using sharp needles. Permanent damage of nerves and other structures is rare.

5.9 Irregularities in the Donor Area

Although more common in the case of aggressive liposuction in which large amounts of fat are obtained, irregularities may occur in cases of facial fat grafting even though the volume required is usually small. It is useful to regularize the donor area with a flat cannula so as to minimize these irregularities.

References

1. Yoshimura K, Coleman SR. Complications of fat grafting: how they occur and how to find, avoid, and treat them. Clin Plast Surg. 2015;42:383–8.
2. Coleman SR. Structural fat grafting: more than a permanent filler. Plast Reconstr Surg. 2006;118(3 Suppl):108S–20.
3. Tonnard P, Verpaele A, Peeters G, Hamdi M, Cornelissen M, Declercq H. Nanofat grafting: basic research and clinical applications. Plast Reconstr Surg. 2013;132:1017–26.
4. Paik JS, Cho WK, Park GS, Yang SW. Eyelid-associated complications after autogenous fat injection for cosmetic forehead augmentation. BMC Ophthalmol. 2013;13:32.
5. Serra-Mestre JM, Serra-Renom JM, Martinez L, Almadori A, D'Andrea F. Platelet-rich plasma mixed-fat grafting: a reasonable prosurvival strategy for fat grafts? Aesthetic Plast Surg. 2014;38:1041–9.
6. Fontdevila J, Serra-Renom JM, Raigosa M, Berenguer J, Guisantes E, Prades E, et al. Assessing the long-term viability of facial fat grafts: an objective measure using computed tomography. Aesthet Surg J. 2008;28:380–6.
7. Coleman SR, Katzel EB. Fat grafting for facial filling and regeneration. Clin Plast Surg. 2015;42:289–300.
8. Zhu M, Xie Y, Zhu Y, Chai G, Li Q. A novel noninvasive three-dimensional volumetric analysis for fat-graft survival in facial recontouring using the 3L and 3M technique. J Plast Reconstr Aesthet Surg. 2016;69(2):248–54.
9. Egido JA, Arroyo R, Marcos A, Jiménez-Alfaro I. Middle cerebral artery embolism and unilateral visual loss after autologous fat injection into the glabellar area. Stroke. 1993;24:615–6.
10. Danesh-Meyer HV, Savino PJ, Sergott RC. Case reports and small case series: ocular and cerebral ischemia following facial injection of autologous fat. Arch Ophthalmol. 2001;119:777–8.
11. Sherman JE, Fanzio PM, White H, Leifer D. Blindness and necrotizing fasciitis after liposuction and fat transfer. Plast Reconstr Surg. 2010;126:1358–63.
12. Park YH, Kim KS. Images in clinical medicine. Blindness after fat injections. N Engl J Med. 2011;365:2220.
13. Hong DK, Seo YJ, Lee JH, Im M. Sudden visual loss and multiple cerebral infarction after autologous fat injection into the glabella. Dermatol Surg. 2014;40:485–7.

A How-to Guide on Structural Fat Grafting, Microfat Grafting, Sharp-Needle Intradermal Fat, Nanofat Grafting, and Emulsion or Fractioned Fat

6

Depending on the fat graft required, certain modifications are necessary during the fat preparation, processing, and injection. This is especially true in the facial region, where the use of different sizes of fat grafts and the combination of deep injections with a cannula and superficial injections with a needle have improved results—not only in correcting volume depletions but in cases of fine remodeling, as well.

Below we provide a step-by-step explanation of the preparation of each of the different fat grafts.

6.1 Donor Site Selection

When we need fat for grafting, we weigh up the different possible donor sites and choose the most suitable with the agreement with the patient.

It is very important not to create irregularities in the donor sites; a good cosmetic result must be achieved in the area to be grafted, but the most commonly used areas in our practice for facial fat grafting are first the abdomen, the inner thigh, and the inside of the knee and then the flanks, the hips, and if necessary, the back of the thigh (Fig. 6.1).

6.1.1 Abdomen

The part of the abdomen most commonly used as a donor site is the subumbilical area. Many patients have a sufficient amount of adipose tissue here; however, several points need to be kept in mind. The first is the fact that the fat above and below the Scarpa fascia differs considerably. Second it is easy to leave irregularities; we cannot perform fat grafting to improve one area of the body but leave the abdomen disfigured.

When small amounts are needed, we enter via the navel; when greater quantities are required, we make two additional lateral incisions so that we can cross the tunnels and make sure that there are no irregularities after obtaining the abdominal fat required (Fig. 6.2a). With a flat 3-mm cannula without aspiration, we regularize the whole area where the fat was harvested and remove any depressions (Fig. 6.2b).

6.1.2 Flank

Sometimes when the abdomen is chosen as the donor site, we find that more fat is required. In this case, fat can be easily obtained from the flanks (provided that the patient has sufficient quantities) using the same lateral incision as the one used in the abdomen (Fig. 6.3).

6.1.3 Inner Thigh

In thin patients with insufficient abdominal fat, the amounts needed can be obtained from the inside of the thigh (Fig. 6.4). If performed correctly and if the incision is hidden in the groin fold, the area regularizes very well. Patients tend to be very happy and do not mind having lost some volume in this area, but great care must be taken not to leave irregularities.

© Springer International Publishing Switzerland 2016
J.M. Serra-Renom, J.M. Serra-Mestre, *Atlas of Minimally Invasive Facelift*, DOI 10.1007/978-3-319-33018-1_6

6.1.4   Hip

The hip is in a very convenient location and provides good volume. Before extraction, the patient is shown where the incisions will be made. Extraction is possible only with one incision, but we prefer to make two and to cross the tunnels above and below the site where the fat is obtained (Fig. 6.5).

6.1.5   Back of the Thigh

Sometimes it is necessary to remove fat from more areas, if, for example, more volume is needed or if no fat is available in the usual sites. In these cases we use the back of the thigh (Fig. 6.6). This is also a useful area, but the disadvantage is that the patient has to be turned over.

6.1.6   Inner Side of the Knee

The inner side of the knee is a frequently used donor site especially in young, thin women because it is an area where there is always a small accumulation of fat in women (though not in men).

To obtain fat, after creating the tumescence, we pinch the skin and obtain fat with a multiperforated cannula (Fig. 6.7).

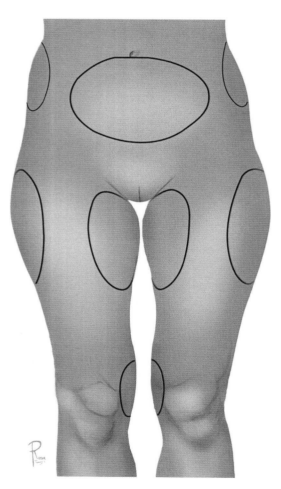

Fig. 6.1 Donor sites

Fig. 6.2 (**a**) Abdominal liposuction. (**b**) Regularization of the donor site using a 3-mm flat cannula without aspiration

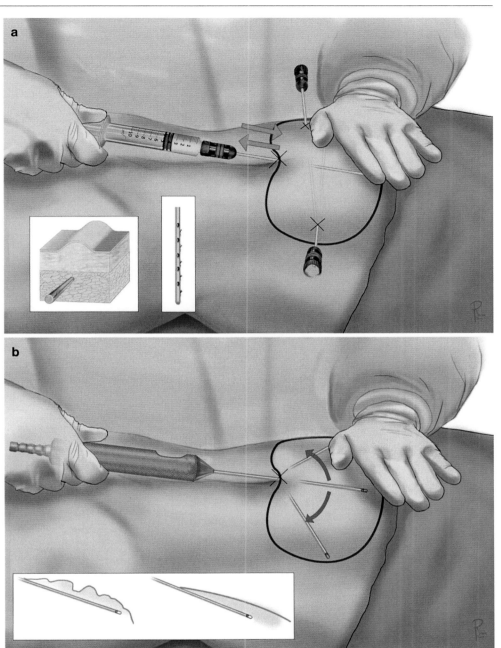

Fig. 6.3 Flanks: Sufficient liposuction can be performed without changing the patient's position

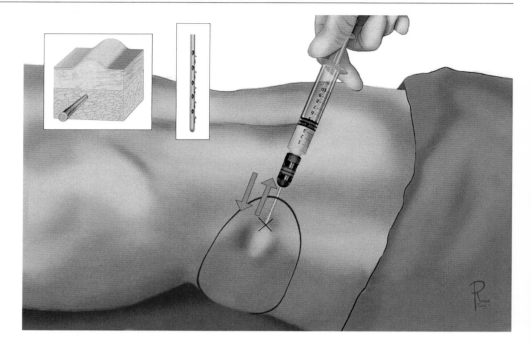

Fig. 6.4 Inner thigh

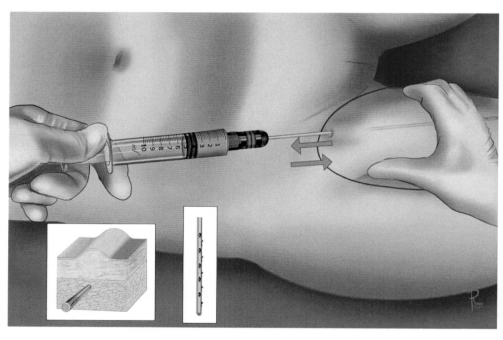

Fig. 6.5 The hip

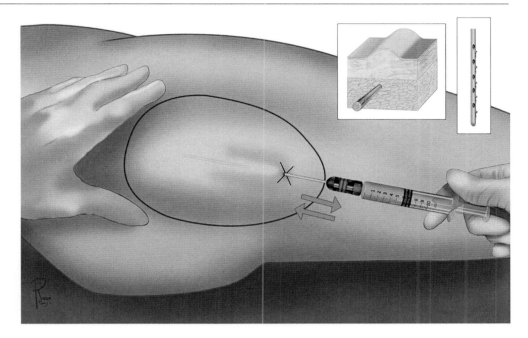

Fig. 6.6 Back of the thigh

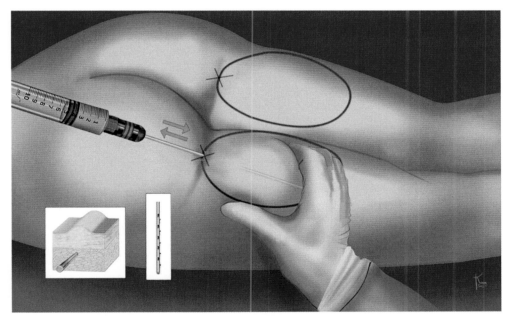

Fig. 6.7 Inside of the knee

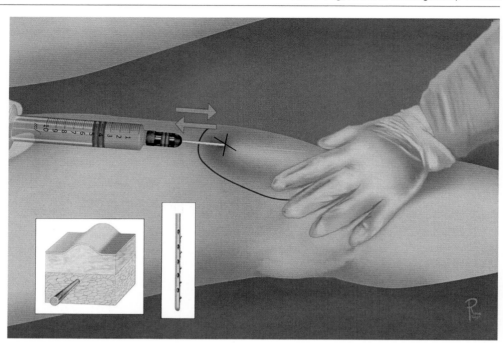

6.2   **Fat Harvesting**

After selecting the donor area, first the tumescence is created with a multiperforated blunt cannula. When surgery is performed under local anesthesia, the tumescent solution contains 0.05 % lidocaine in saline solution and 1: 200,000 epinephrine. When the procedure is performed under general anesthetic, the tumescence can be done with a vasoconstrictor alone diluted in saline solution or by adding low concentrations of local anesthetic (0.02 % lidocaine). After tumescence, we wait around 20 min before starting liposuction.

The aspiration pressure can be generated either with handheld syringe aspiration or with the liposuctor at a low pressure, around 0.5 atm.

To obtain structural fat grafting, a 3-mm cannula is used. If the aim is to obtain microfat grafts, whether they are to be injected via a cannula or a needle (in the case of sharp-needle intradermal fat grafts [SNIF]), nanofat grafts and emulsion or fractioned fat grafts, 2.4-mm microport harvester cannulas with barbed and beveled 1-mm ports are very useful. Once we have obtained the fat, it is placed on a grid (Fig. 6.8).

Fig. 6.8 Fat harvesting

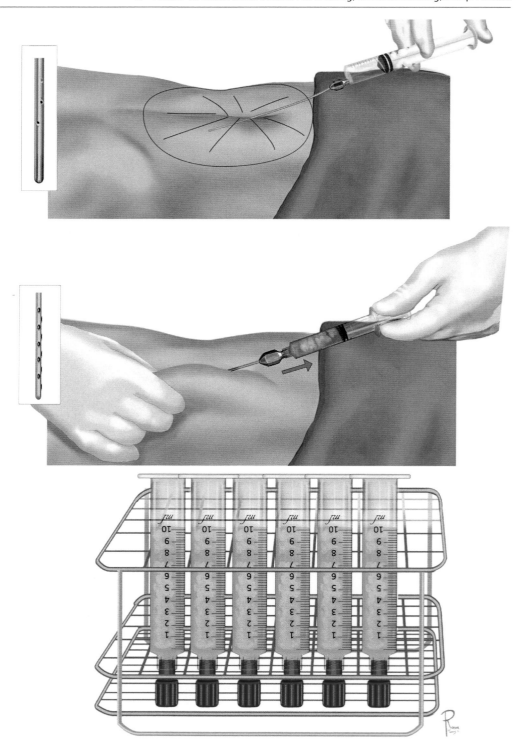

6.3 Fat Processing Techniques and Injection

6.3.1 Structural Fat Grafting

As discussed in Chap. 3, a variety of methods can be used to isolate the fat from other components of the aspirated material. Although there is no general agreement as yet on the method that achieves the best results and causes the least cell damage, in our clinical practice, we use centrifugation, filtration, and decanting interchangeably for structural fat grafting and have obtained similar results.

In the case of centrifugation, we use an oblique centrifuge for 2 min at 2000 rpm. Once centrifuged, three levels can be observed in the syringes. The lower level contains blood and debris, water, and components of the tumescence solution; the middle layer consists of small lipomas; and the top layer contains oil resulting from the broken down fatty acids. We discard the bottom layer of anesthetic and blood and then remove the upper part containing the fat droplets with a small gauze (Fig. 6.9a).

We then connect the 10-mL syringe with the clean fat to a connector or a three-way stopcock to a 1- or 2-mL syringe and transfer the fat. We connect the syringe to a 1.6-mm cannula and perform the fat grafting (Fig. 6.9b) [1].

6.3.2 Microfat Grafting and Sharp-Needle Intradermal Fat (SNIF)

Our decanting and washing technique has given us very good results, since it is a closed method and the fat obtained is very clean. First, we aspirate the fat with a 10-mL syringe, creating a vacuum with the syringe and a Tulip cannula.

After this, we fill only half of the syringe, i.e., 5 mL. We then fill the syringe up to 9 mL with 4 mL of Ringer lactate. We withdraw the embolus of the syringe 1 mL to create a space.

Now that we have this space, we shake the syringe a little to clean the fat and then leave it standing vertically for a few minutes. Within a few minutes, some very yellow fat appears floating on the surface; below are the remains of the blood and the anesthetic. If it is not sufficiently clean, we empty this transparent lower part and aspirate 4 mL of Ringer lactate, shake it again, and decant it so that it is thoroughly cleaned. We then empty the lower level and transfer the purified fat to a 1-mL syringe for injection (Fig. 6.10a).

For injection of the microfat graft, we use cannulas smaller than 1 mm in diameter (usually around 0.7 mm). The choice of a straight or curved blunt cannula depends on the defect to be treated. The injection is made in the subcutaneous plane (Fig. 6.10b) [2].

When this fat is injected into more superficial planes, as in the case of SNIF, 23-G sharp needles [3] are used.

6.3.3 Emulsion, Fractioned Fat and Sharp-Needle Intradermal Emulsion (SNIE)

Once the fat has been obtained and washed, we take a syringe with 5 mL of fat and via a three-way stopcock connect it to an empty 10-cm syringe. We transfer the fat from one syringe to the other at least 30 or 40 times. It becomes increasingly liquefied, and there are fewer lipomas; gradually the emulsion is formed (Fig. 6.11a).

Once the fat is well emulsified, we wash it again to remove fatty acids and then aspirate 4 mL of Ringer lactate with the syringe containing the emulsion and shake well. We then decant the emulsion again, and, although more transparent, two layers are now visible: the emulsion on top and the washing liquid on the bottom. We discard the washing liquid and transfer the emulsion to a 1- or 2-mL syringe.

We inject this emulsion either with cannulas of 0.5 mm in diameter to perform filling of the tear trough, for example, or with a 25-G needle (SNIE) in the case of mesotherapy (Fig. 6.11b). The cell counter indicates that the emulsion has a similar number of stromal vascular fraction cells as the nanofat [4].

6.3.4 Nanofat Grafting

To create the nanofat, as described by Tonnard et al. [4], we prepare an emulsion and then filter it through a cloth or grid with 0.5-mm pores or holes.

In this way the collagen fibers and the remains of the membranes remain at the top and a liquid at the bottom, the nanofat. The nanofat is aspirated with a 2-mL syringe and transferred via a three-way stopcock to a 1-mL syringe; it is then connected to a 27-G needle and injected into the dermis (Fig. 6.12) [4]. This highly liquid preparation is very useful, for example, for improving the color of the region beneath the eyes. The cell counter indicates that the nanofat has the same number of stromal vascular fraction cells as the emulsion.

a

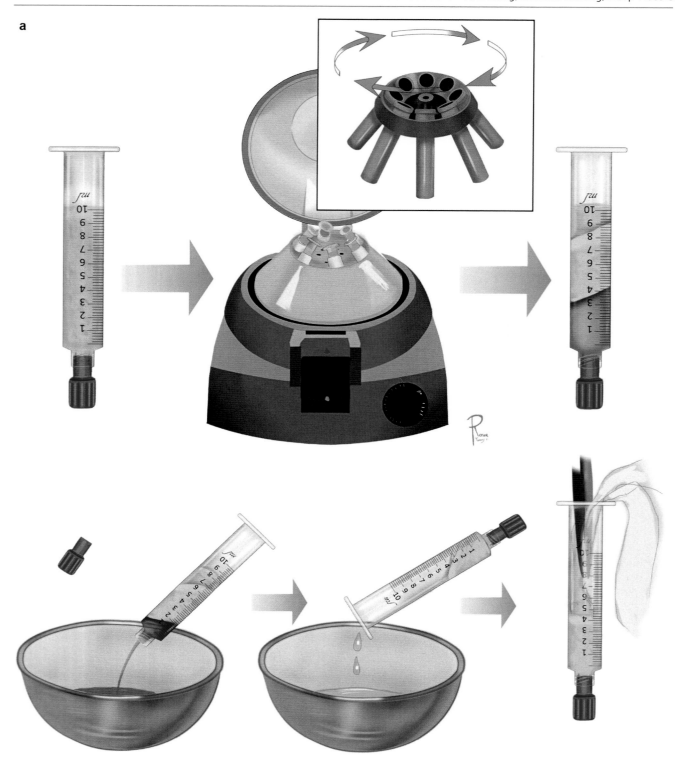

Fig. 6.9 Centrifugation. (**a**) The three levels that appear after centrifugation; isolation of the fat. (**b**) The fat is transferred to smaller volume syringes for injection, which is performed with a cannula in the subcutaneous plane

Fig. 6.9 (continued)

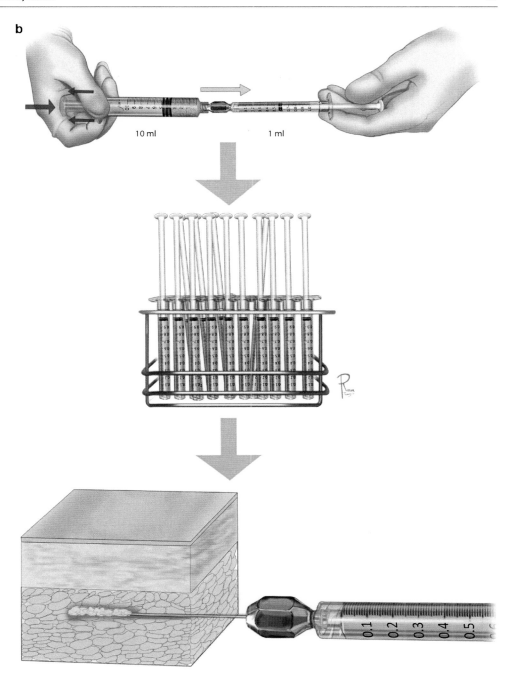

10 ml   1 ml

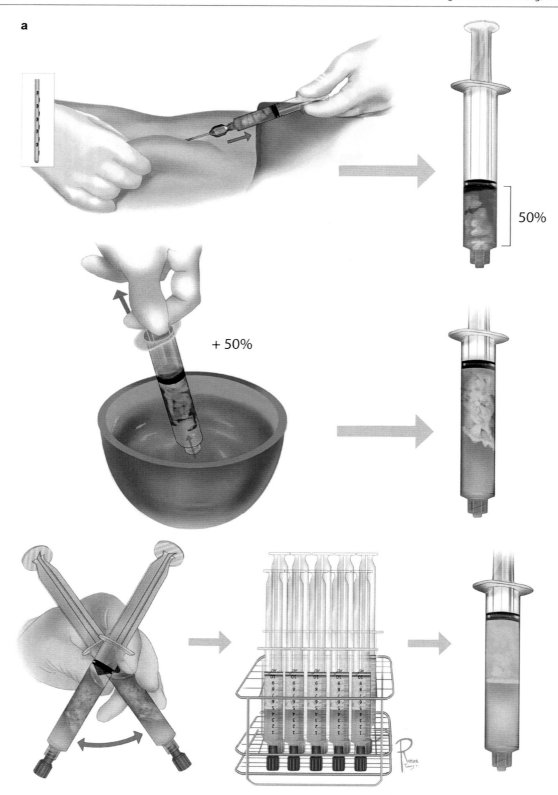

Fig. 6.10 Decanting and washing technique. (**a**) A quick and simple method for washing and decanting the fat by filling each syringe with a mixture of 50 % fat and 50 % saline solution. (**b**) This method is used for microfat grafting and SNIF, since the fat obtained with the centrifugation is more compact and is more likely to cause obstruction in small cannulas or syringes

b

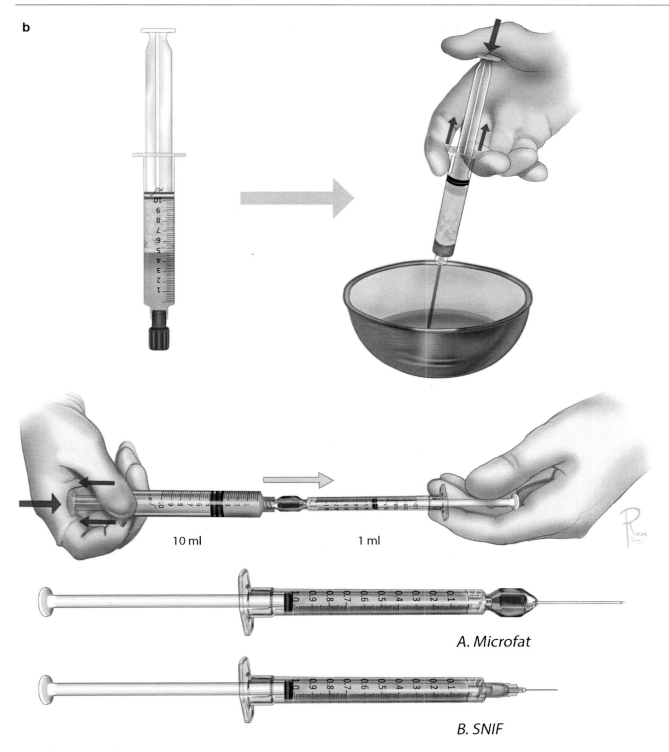

10 ml   1 ml

A. Microfat

B. SNIF

Fig. 6.10 (continued)

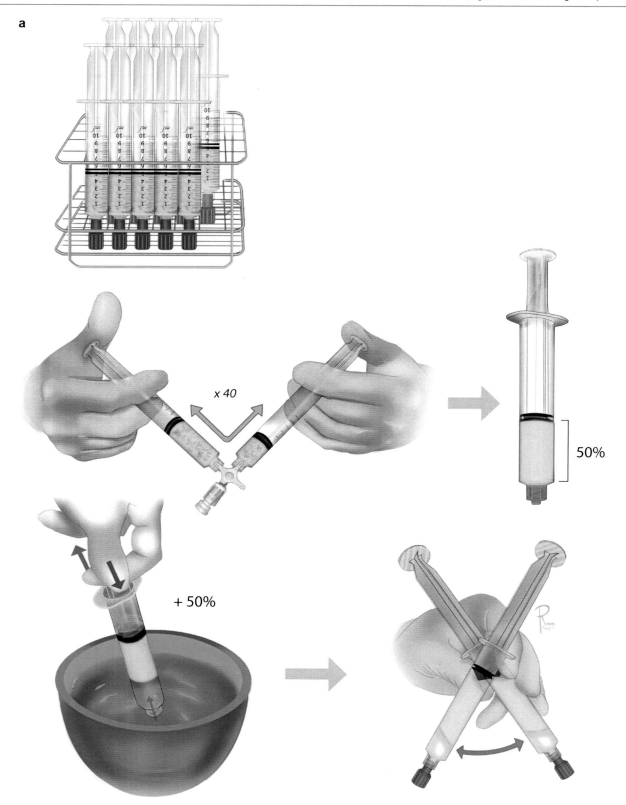

Fig. 6.11 Emulsion or fractioned fat. (**a**) A mechanical emulsion of microfat grafts is made in two syringes and then washed and decanted. (**b**) The injection can be performed with either a cannula (emulsion or fractioned fat) or a syringe (SNIE, which refers to Sharp Needle Intradermal Emulsion)

b

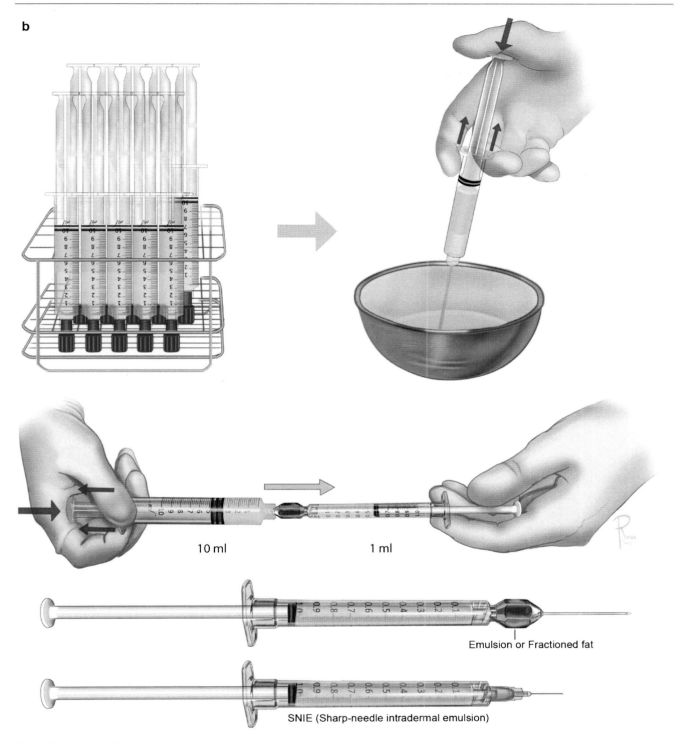

10 ml   1 ml

Emulsion or Fractioned fat

SNIE (Sharp-needle intradermal emulsion)

Fig. 6.11 (continued)

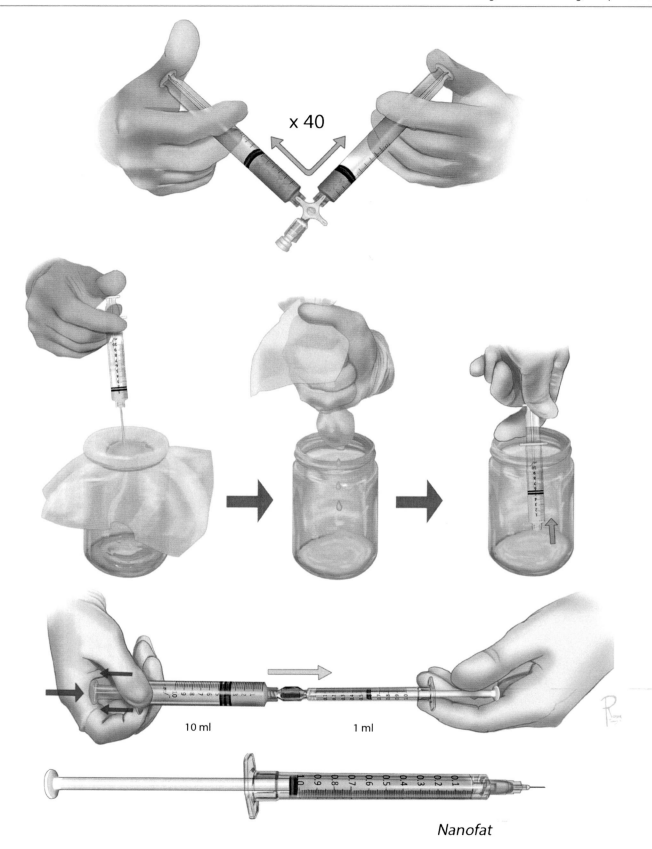

Fig. 6.12 Nanofat graft: a mechanical emulsion is made and then filtered. The liquid resulting after filtration is known as nanofat. It is injected with 27-G needles

6.4   The Use of Platelet Growth Factors in Facial Rejuvenation

To obtain the platelets, it is very important to use an oscillating rotor to ensure that the tubes containing blood remain completely horizontal after spinning in the centrifuge. If an oblique or vertical rotor is used, the platelets are impacted with the red blood cells, and none remain in the upper part of the tube.

When extracting the blood, it is important to ensure that the needle does not damage the vessel because otherwise it will be cloudy and the platelets will not be separated after centrifugation. Using a needle placed in a vein, we aspirate with a blood collection tube already containing the citrate. We can also use a 20-mL syringe and add 2 mL of sodium citrate.

This mixture is shaken and placed in the oscillating centrifuge for 8 min at 1800 rpm (Fig. 6.13a). After this, three levels appear: the top level with platelets and plasma; then a very thin, darker middle level with leukocytes that should not be aspirated because it might increase the inflammatory reaction; and finally the bottom level with the red blood cells.

Once the platelets are obtained, the tube is placed upright in the rack. The top third of the platelets comprise the plasma poor in growth factor (PPGF); the middle third, the plasma growth factor (PGF) with the same concentration of platelets as in the blood; and the bottom third, the plasma rich in growth factor (PRGF). Then with a pipette we separate the platelets from the rest. If we want to obtain PRGF we discard the upper two-thirds. If we want to use the platelets as anti-inflammatory agents in the area where the mesotherapy is to be performed, we use the entire platelet concentration (Fig. 6.13b).

After obtaining the platelets, they are stimulated before the mixtures are made. This is done with calcium chloride in a ratio of 1:20, i.e., 1 mL of calcium chloride is added to 20 mL of platelets.

If we want to perform mesotherapy, it is important to act swiftly; once the platelets are stimulated with calcium chloride, they form a gel, and then the solution cannot be injected. If this process is omitted, the platelets nevertheless become stimulated once inside the body.

The platelets can be mixed with the microfat, the emulsion, or also with the nanofat. When we want to perform mesotherapy, we mix them with the emulsion or nanofat. They can also be mixed with vitamins; i.e., the mixture may contain only the anti-inflammatory platelets we use in facelifts or platelets plus emulsion in the case of mesotherapy. When we perform mesotherapy and require only a small amount, we use the PRGF fraction and sometimes add vitamins to the mixture. Therefore, the choice of mixture depends on the needs of each patient (Fig. 6.13c).

In facelifts, we use platelets throughout the detached area as anti-inflammatory and sealing agents.

In mesotherapy with highly damaged skin, we use platelets with vitamins.

To fill the malar region, nasolabial folds, and marionette lines, we use platelets together with emulsion or microfat [5].

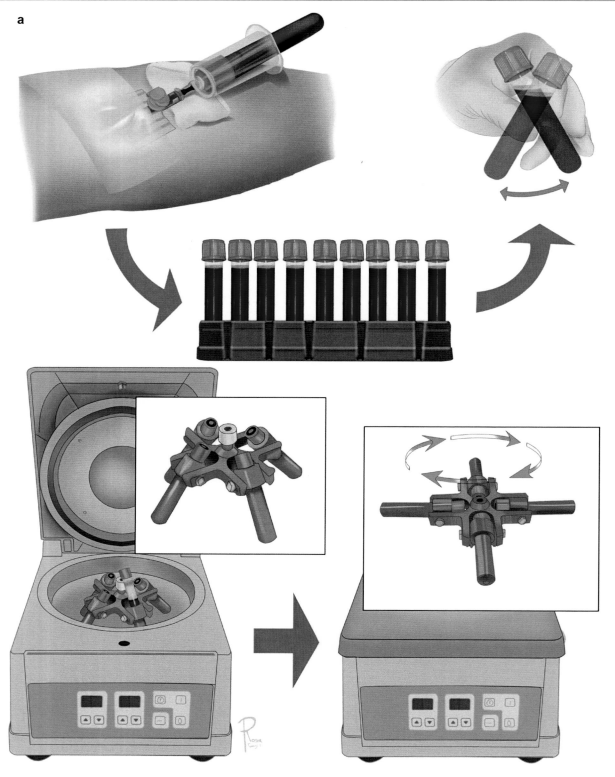

Fig. 6.13 Platelet growth factors. (**a**) Blood is obtained with citrate tubes and centrifuged in an oscillating centrifuge. (**b**) The three levels after centrifugation. For the degranulation of platelet alpha granules, activation is necessary. (**c**) It can be combined with fat, emulsion, nanofat, or vitamins for joint injection

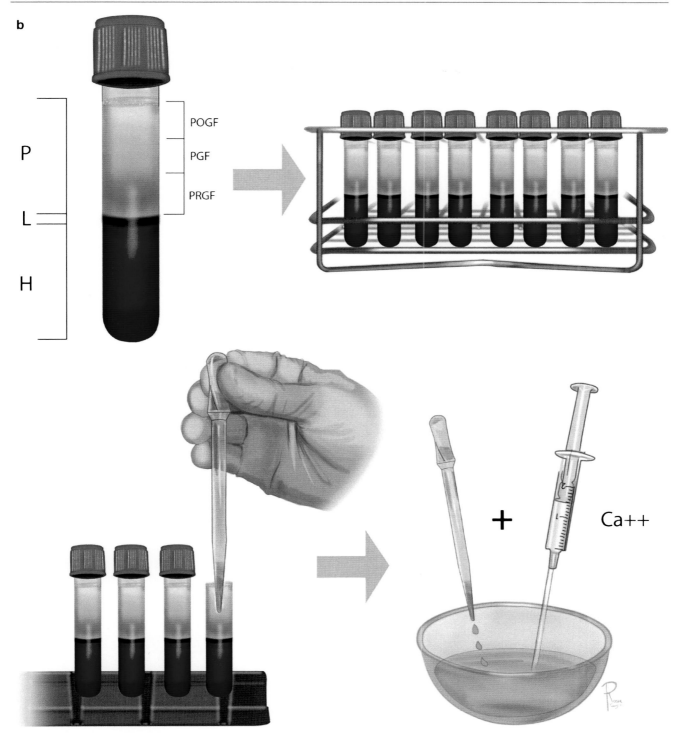

Fig. 6.13 (continued)

c

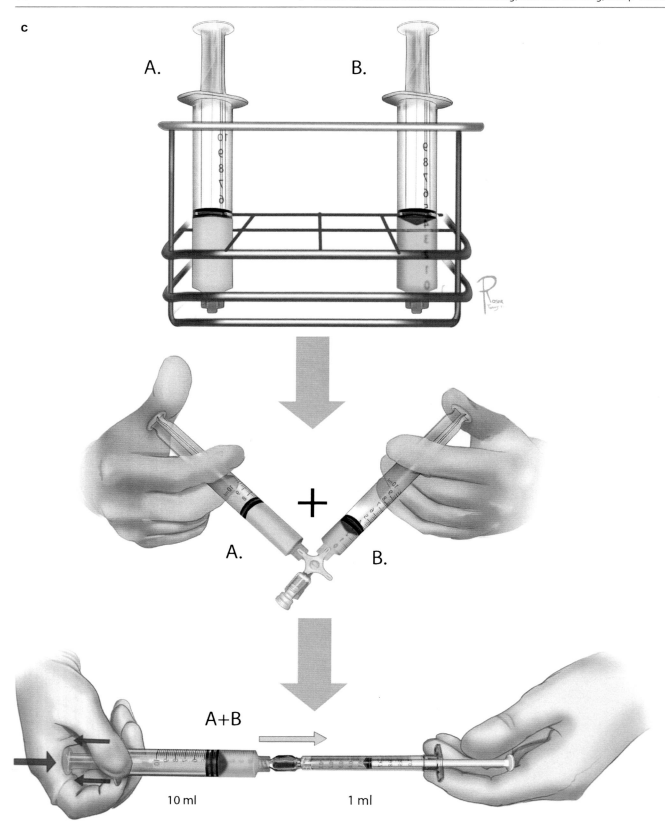

A.

B.

+

A.

B.

A+B

10 ml

1 ml

Fig. 6.13 (continued)

References

1. Coleman SR. Facial augmentation with structural fat grafting. Clin Plast Surg. 2006;33:567–77.
2. Lindenblatt N, van Hulle A, Verpaele AM, Tonnard PL. The role of microfat grafting in facial contouring. Aesthet Surg J. 2015;35:763–71.
3. Zeltzer AA, Tonnard PL, Verpaele AM. Sharp-needle intradermal fat grafting (SNIF). Aesthet Surg J. 2012;32:554–61.
4. Tonnard P, Verpaele A, Peeters G, Hamdi M, Cornelissen M, Declercq H. Nanofat grafting: basic research and clinical applications. Plast Reconstr Surg. 2013;132:1017–26.
5. Serra-Mestre JM, Serra-Renom JM, Martinez L, Almadori A, D'Andrea F. Platelet-rich plasma mixed-fat grafting: a reasonable prosurvival strategy for fat grafts? Aesthetic Plast Surg. 2014;38:1041–9.

Facial Fat Grafting

To obtain the most natural-looking results possible, it is necessary to reestablish a rejuvenated facial contour, complementing conventional approaches that can correct excess skin laxity with procedures to provide volume at the points where it has been lost.

Relevant superficial and deep fat compartments separated from each other by connective tissue membranes that stabilize the perforator blood supply to the skin must be considered when volume replacement is performed in order to achieve an accurate facial volumization [1].

With regard to the superficial compartments, the nasolabial fat (NLF) and superficial medial cheek (SMC) fat compartments primarily form the central region of the face. Superior to the SMC and above the orbicularis, the infraorbital fat compartment is located, which seems to have a poor lymphatic drainage. Lateral to the lateral canthus, there is the middle superficial cheek and lateral temporal compartments.

Deep compartments comprise the suborbicularis oculi fat (SOOF), which has a medial and a lateral component and lies deep to the orbicularis oculi muscle of the lower lid and superficial to the dense posterior capsule of the superficial muscular aponeurotic system (SMAS) enveloping the orbicularis oculi. In the midface the deep medial cheek (DMC) fat compartment, divided into a medial unit located deep and medial to the nasolabial fat and a lateral part (DLC), which is found deep to the SMC, is probably the most important compartment when improvement of the anterior cheek projection is desired. When filling this compartment, it is advisable to avoid placing the fat too lateral to avoid migration into the buccal recess. The buccal extension of the buccal fat pad is located just lateral to the DLC [1–3].

In the next chapters, we will describe the areas where facial fat grafting is performed in topographic order from the forehead to the neck (Fig. 7.1).

© Springer International Publishing Switzerland 2016
J.M. Serra-Renom, J.M. Serra-Mestre, *Atlas of Minimally Invasive Facelift*, DOI 10.1007/978-3-319-33018-1_7

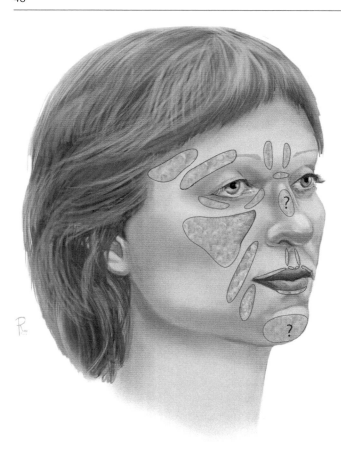

Fig. 7.1 Areas in which facial fat grafting are used. The "?" sign refers to those areas where its injection is not common but can be useful in selected cases and associated with rhinoplasty

References

1. Rohrich RJ, Pessa JE. The fat compartments of the face: anatomy and clinical implications for cosmetic surgery. Plast Reconstr Surg. 2007;119:2219–27; discussion 2228–31.
2. Gierloff M, Stöhring C, Buder T, Wiltfang J. The subcutaneous fat compartments in relation to aesthetically important facial folds and rhytides. J Plast Reconstr Aesthet Surg. 2012;65:1292–7.
3. Surek CC, Beut J, Stephens R, Jelks G, Lamb J. Pertinent anatomy and analysis for midface volumizing procedures. Plast Reconstr Surg. 2015;135:818e–29.

Frontal, Temple, and Periorbital Fat Grafting

Volumetric rejuvenation of the periorbital region and the upper third of the face has two applications. First, it is a useful technique for filling and correcting the various kinds of wrinkles that appear during aging in this area, which is one of the most frequently treated problems. Fat is one of a number of fillers used and gives good results.

Second, fat injection is revolutionizing periorbital rejuvenation, understood to include not just the removal of excess skin and eyelid fat pads with blepharoplasty but also the correction of volume loss throughout the periorbital area and the improvement of the transition to neighboring areas such as the malar region, the forehead, and the temple.

8.1 Glabellar Frown Lines

Glabellar wrinkles can be subdivided as follows: vertical, when caused by hyperactivity of the transverse head of the corrugator muscle; horizontal, when located in the nasal root, mainly due to hyperactivity of the procerus muscle; and oblique, when formed by the oblique portion of the corrugator muscle and also by the depressor supercilii muscle [1, 2].

Before fat grafting, it is advisable to correct the hyperactivity of these muscles. This can be done by injecting botulinum toxin 10 days before surgery [3] or by transpalpebral resection of the corrugator and procerus muscles using the blepharoplasty incision in the upper eyelid [4].

The vertical frown lines are treated with a subcutaneous injection of fat using the sharp-needle intradermal fat graft (SNIF) technique. The entry point is the upper part of the frown line. The amount of fat to be injected ranges between 0.5 and 1 mL on either side (Fig. 8.1a). We then give an intradermal injection from the other end of the line using SNIF (Fig. 8.1b). If this does not remove the line, we introduce small vertical injections of emulsion into the dermis above it (Fig. 8.1c). After treating the two vertical frown lines, we regularize the glabellar area, treating the horizontal lines at the nasal root and in the intermediate zone by subcutaneous SNIF until the whole of the glabellar area and nasal root are corrected.

J.M. Serra-Renom, J.M. Serra-Mestre, *Atlas of Minimally Invasive Facelift*, DOI 10.1007/978-3-319-33018-1_8

Fig. 8.1 Glabellar frown lines.
(**a**) Subcutaneous injection with
SNIF. (**b**) Intradermal injection
with SNIF. (**c**) Vertical injections
of emulsion into the dermis
(SNIE)

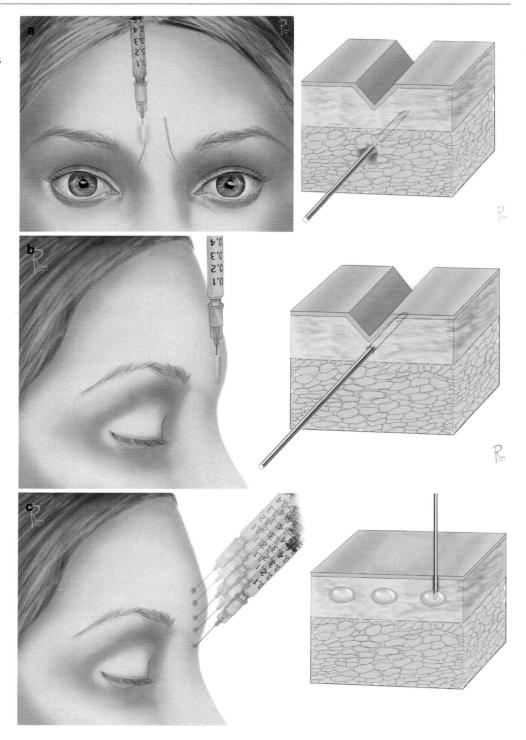

8.2   Tail of the Eyebrow

To reshape the orbital rim and slightly raise the tail of the eyebrow, first we mark the supraorbital nerve located at the point where, following a straight ascending vertical line from the pupil, it intersects the eyebrow [2]; we also identify the area to be injected in the shape of an ellipse along the orbital rim bone by palpation.

First, we make a puncture with an Abbocath catheter no. 16; then we inject subcutaneous microfat with a cannula throughout the area until we are satisfied with the appearance. In this way, with the injection of approximately 1 mL of fat, we obtain a good remodeling of the tail of the eyebrow (Fig. 8.2).

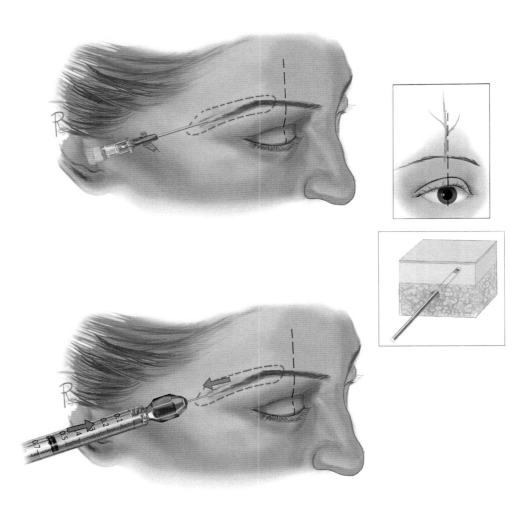

Fig. 8.2 Tail of the eyebrow. *Above*, puncture with Abbocath. Observe the markings performed in previous injection; *below*, injection of microfat with a blunt cannula

8.3   Temporal Region

We sometimes perform fat injections in the temporal region using microfat. We insert a 16G Abbocath catheter and then perform a subcutaneous injection with a cannula

after aspiration and distribute the fat evenly, taking great care not to damage any of the veins (Fig. 8.3).

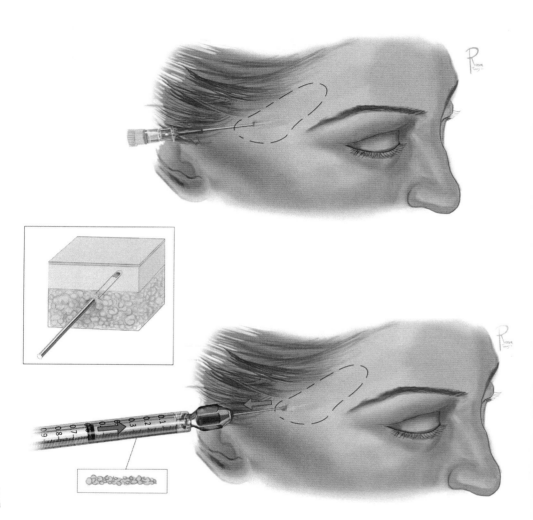

Fig. 8.3 Temporal region.
Above, puncture with Abbocath;
below, injection of microfat with
a blunt cannula

8.4 Injection for Crow's Feet in External Orbital Rim

To treat crow's feet appearing on the outer edge of the eye, first we inject microfat with a cannula along the entire orbital rim (Fig. 8.4a).

We then perform SNIF using a needle in the dermal-subdermal plane in each of the wrinkles in fan-shaped tunnels (Fig. 8.4b).

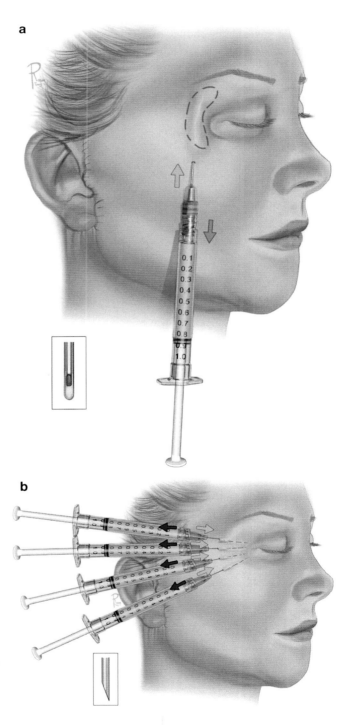

Fig. 8.4 (**a**) To treat crow's feet appearing on the outer edge of the eye, first we inject microfat with a cannula. (**b**) SNIF is also performed in each of the wrinkles

8.5   Tear Trough

The nasojugal groove or tear trough is the groove on the inner edge of the eye running downward and oblique from the lacrimal caruncle between the levator ala of the nose and the orbicularis muscle (Fig. 8.5a).

To treat the tear trough, we infuse emulsion via a cannula. At about 2 cm from the lacrimal caruncle (in the tear trough, at the most distal vertex), we insert an Abbocath catheter and then use a fine cannula to inject emulsion, filling the entire

tear trough in a downward direction. Great care is needed, and only a very small amount of emulsion should be injected—usually between 0.2 and 0.4 mL. After injecting this emulsion into the subcutaneous plane, we gently flatten it with the finger.

If the skin is dark in color, first we inject nanofat [5] into the dermis above the tear trough in very small amounts (Fig. 8.5b). We then flatten it gently with the finger (Fig. 8.5c) and inject the emulsion in a subcutaneous plane if required (Fig. 8.5d).

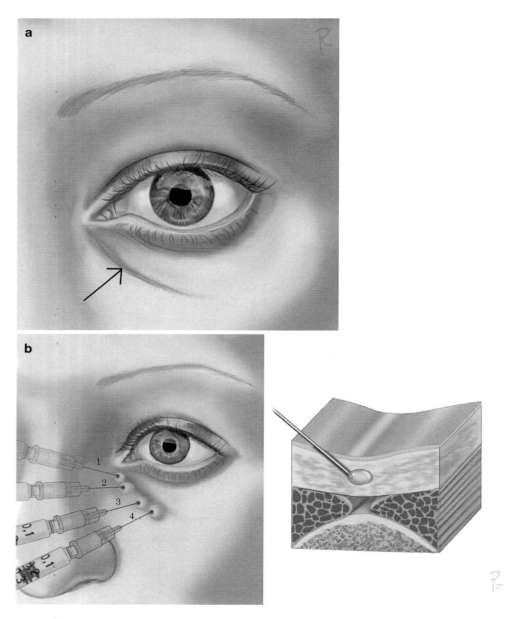

Fig. 8.5 Tear trough. (**a**) Location of the tear trough. (**b**) If the skin is dark, nanofat or SNIE is perfomed. (**c**) After injecting nanofat, it is convenient to flatten the injected zones gently with the finger.

(**d**) Correction of volume depletions in this area is performed with microfat or emulsion injection using a blunt fine cannula

Fig. 8.5 (continued)

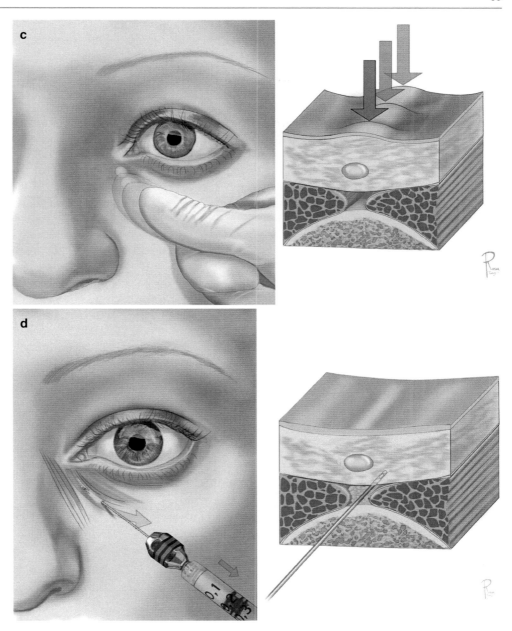

8.6 Treatment of the Hollowing and Herniation of Lower Eyelid Fat Pads and Dark Circles Under the Eyes

Patients want to remove the excess fat under their eyes, but they also want to avoid the appearance of sunken or dark circles (Fig. 8.6a). To achieve this, we first prefer to perform the lower blepharoplasty by a transconjunctival approach (Fig. 8.6b, c) [6, 7]. In necessary cases, although we favor the treatment of the excess skin of the lower eyelid very conservatively, we perform peeling with trichloroacetic acid or with a minimal resection of the skin without resecting the orbicular muscle, using the skin pinching technique; this allows us to leave the middle lamella intact and reduces the chance of scleral show or ectropion [8].

After this correction, we assess the height of the eyelid, which may remain excessively long and may give an appearance of tiredness, even though the fat herniation has been addressed. We now perform fat grafting around the orbital rim to reduce the height of the lower eyelid.

With the aid of a cannula and with microfat, we perform a small fat grafting in the orbital rim in a downward direction. It is very important not to use microfat in the eyelid in order to avoid irregularities but to use it in the part of the orbital rim toward the cheekbone. We then extract the cannula and insert a syringe with a cannula and emulsion; we gently introduce the emulsion from the orbital rim upward in the region of the eyelid that is slightly sunken, so that it remains flat and joins together with the fat we have injected into the orbital rim (Fig. 8.6d, e). Thus, with the mixture of emulsion and microfat, we correct the height of the lower eyelid and improve the skin color. We continue with microfat grafting in the malar area if it is necessary to correct the negative vector.

The amounts of fat grafted in the orbital region are microfat from the orbital rim downward in the malar region 0.5–1 mL and emulsion from the orbital rim upward 0.3–0.5 mL.

If the skin under the eye is dark, we can improve the color by injecting nanofat into the dermis in very small amounts (maximum 0.3 or 0.4 mL) using a 27-G needle (Fig. 8.6f). We gently flatten it with the finger until the irregularities disappear. This must be done before injecting fat in the deep plane, because in this case the massaging would displace the fat injected deep beneath the surface.

Fig. 8.6 Blepharoplasty and fat grafting. (**a**) Most frequent aging pattern of the lower eyelid. (**b**) Release of the arcus marginalis helps to improve dark circles under the eyes. (**c**) Transconjuntival blepharoplasty. (**d**) Emulsion is injected from the orbital rim upward in the region of the eyelid. (**e**) Microfat in the orbital rim and malar area in order to improve the transition between these areas. (**f**) Injection of nanofat or SNIE to improve the color of the skin in the lower eyelid

Fig. 8.6 (continued)

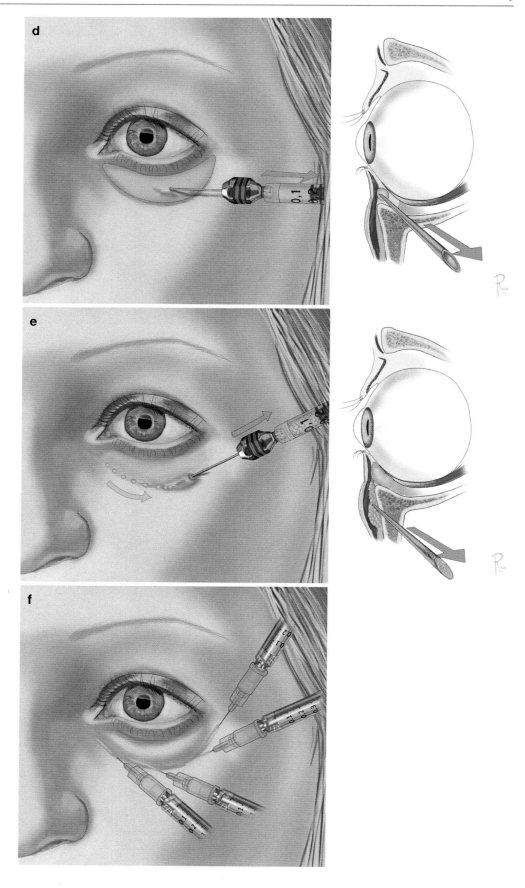

References

1. Janis JE, Ghavami A, Lemmon JA, Leedy JE, Guyuron B. Anatomy of the corrugator supercilii muscle: part I. Corrugator topography. Plast Reconstr Surg. 2007;120:1647–53.
2. Janis JE, Ghavami A, Lemmon JA, Leedy JE, Guyuron B. The anatomy of the corrugator supercilii muscle: part II. Supraorbital nerve branching patterns. Plast Reconstr Surg. 2008;121:233–40.
3. Bassichis BA, Thomas JR. The use of Botox to treat glabellar rhytids. Facial Plast Surg Clin North Am. 2005;13:11–4.
4. Knize DM. Transpalpebral approach to the corrugator supercilii and procerus muscles. Plast Reconstr Surg. 1995;95:52–60; discussion 61–2.
5. Tonnard P, Verpaele A, Peeters G, et al. Nanofat grafting: basic research and clinical applications. Plast Reconstr Surg. 2013;132:1017–26.
6. Perkins SW, Dyer 2nd WK, Simo F. Transconjunctival approach to lower eyelid blepharoplasty. Experience, indications, and technique in 300 patients. Arch Otolaryngol Head Neck Surg. 1994;120:172–7.
7. Serra-Renom JM, Serra-Mestre JM. Periorbital rejuvenation to improve the negative vector with blepharoplasty and fat grafting in the malar area. Ophthal Plast Reconstr Surg. 2011;27:442–6.
8. Kim EM, Bucky LP. Power of the pinch: pinch lower lid blepharoplasty. Ann Plast Surg. 2008;60:532–7.

Malar Area: Correction of the Facial Negative Vector

In our opinion, the correction of the facial negative vector is one of the most important applications of fat grafting in facial rejuvenation. The term negative vector refers to the ptosis and atrophy of the malar fat compartments, which make the lower lid appear very long when seen in profile and when the angle of the cheek is posterior to the surface of the cornea [1–5].

A young face has a short lower eyelid and a remodeled, full, and curved facial contour anterior to the corneal surface in profile; therefore, when the person is smiling, the malar fat pad rises, giving a more youthful appearance. The most effective way of achieving these features is to convert the negative vector of the upper midface concavity into the positive vector of the upper midface convexity.

Malar fat grafting also helps to make the two cheekbones symmetrical; in fact, it is the only technique that allows us to fully equalize the cheekbones. Thanks to the properties of the fat stromal vascular fraction, the quality of the skin is also improved after injection [4].

9.1 Malar Fat Grafting

For malar fat grafting, we use two entry points. The first is located 2 cm below the external canthus at the level of the zygomatic arch. With a 14-G Abbocath catheter, we create an entry point for the introduction of the Coleman cannula. We make deep fan-shaped tunnels obliquely across the malar region, filling from the orbital rim downward and reaching the outside of the nose and the nasolabial fold. We introduce the cannula and inject as we withdraw it. We use between 5 and 7 mL of microfat from this point.

Then a second entry point is made in the lower part of the nasolabial fold at the level of the oral commissure with a 14G Abbocath catheter directed upward. Then with the Coleman cannula, we create three, four, or five fan-shaped tunnels until the correct shape is obtained (Fig. 9.1). It is very important not to inject microfat into the lower eyelid because of the risk of the formation of cysts [4, 5].

© Springer International Publishing Switzerland 2016
J.M. Serra-Renom, J.M. Serra-Mestre, *Atlas of Minimally Invasive Facelift*, DOI 10.1007/978-3-319-33018-1_9

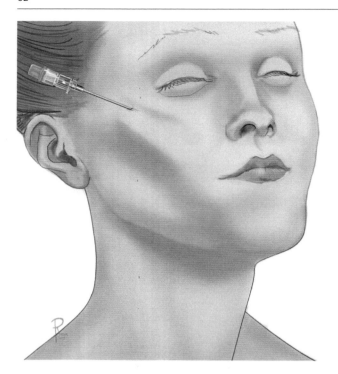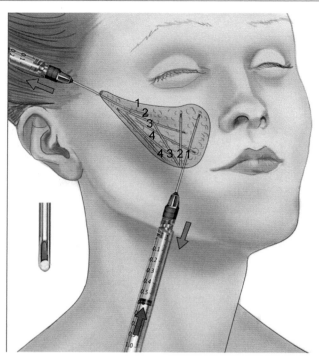

Fig. 9.1   Malar fat grafting with microfat grafting using a blunt cannula. "1–4" refers to the sequence and injection points used when injecting the fat

References

1. Pessa JE, Desvigne LD, Zadoo VP. Changes in ocular globe-to-orbital rim position with age: implications for aesthetic blepharoplasty of the lower eyelids. Aesthetic Plast Surg. 1999;23:337–42.
2. Yaremchuk MJ. Subperiosteal and full-thickness skin rhytidectomy. Plast Reconstr Surg. 2001;107:1045–57.
3. Shaw Jr RB, Katzel EB, Koltz PF, Yaremchuk MJ, Girotto JA, Kahn DM, Langstein HN. Aging of the facial skeleton: aesthetic implications and rejuvenation strategies. Plast Reconstr Surg. 2011;127:374–83.
4. Serra-Renom JM, Serra-Mestre JM. Periorbital rejuvenation to improve the negative vector with blepharoplasty and fat grafting in the malar area. Ophthal Plast Reconstr Surg. 2011;27:442–6.
5. Rohrich RJ, Ghavami A, Constantine FC, Unger J, Mojallal A. Lift-and-fill face lift: integrating the fat compartments. Plast Reconstr Surg. 2014;133:756e–67e.

Nasolabial Folds and Labiomental Creases

Deepening of the nasolabial or labiomental creases is one of the common signs of the aging face. Although lifting techniques can address the gravitational component of these folds, they cannot correct other losses of volume or gravity changes in the older patient, which may notably deepen the nasolabial or labiomental creases around the perioral area [1, 2].

For this reason, these are two of the areas in which a number of different fillers have been used. The choice of filler depends mainly on the depth of the fold, the quality of the skin, and the patient's goals with regard to the permanence of the result.

However, the application of autologous fat grafting in these areas has been less successful than elsewhere. To some extent, this is because injection via a cannula provides volume and improves the aesthetic appearance but is less effective for finer contouring. When using cannulas alone to correct marked folds with a deep, longstanding central wrinkle, we have found that the wrinkle reappeared within a short time even though surgery had been successful. In these cases, attempts to overfill the wrinkle did not obtain entirely satisfactory aesthetic results.

Now, however, we have new forms of microfat injection at our disposal that combine the use of the cannula and fine sharp needles that allow a more superficial injection [3].

The combination of the two injection techniques offers advantages over injection with a cannula alone in a subcutaneous plane. Combining longitudinal injections in the axis of the wrinkle with transverse and perpendicular injections not only enhances the filling of the groove or wrinkle but also prevents the surrounding tissues from folding inward because of lack of support, thus preventing the recurrence of the wrinkle.

10.1 Nasolabial Folds

The entry point where we insert the fine cannula is created with a 14-G Abbocath catheter at the distal end of the nasolabial fold. First, we introduce the cannula until we reach the root of the nasal ala and then inject microfat as we withdraw it. To fill the nasolabial folds, we use from 1 to 2 mL in the subcutaneous plane (Fig. 10.1a). We then inject a sharp-needle intradermal fat graft (SNIF) perpendicular to the nasolabial fold in very shallow intradermal subcutaneous injections, 1 cm long (Fig. 10.1b). In the case of folds with a deep central wrinkle and in which the central line persists after these maneuvers, we perform very gentle intradermal injections of SNIF or SNIE parallel to the fold (Fig. 10.1c).

10.2 Marionette Lines

First we mark the area where the graft is to be performed, following the marionette line or depression. Then, with the aid of a 14-G Abbocath catheter, we place the cannula in an oblique longitudinal direction along the marionette line. We perform fat grafting in two or three subcutaneous tunnels to fill the entire fold with a maximum amount of 1–2 mL. Then, using SNIF, just below the dermis we perform three or four 1-cm-wide intradermal injections perpendicular to the line and parallel to each other, injecting 2 or 3 mL in each in order to fill the depression (Fig. 10.2).

© Springer International Publishing Switzerland 2016
J.M. Serra-Renom, J.M. Serra-Mestre, *Atlas of Minimally Invasive Facelift*, DOI 10.1007/978-3-319-33018-1_10

Fig. 10.1 Nasolabial folds. (**a**)
Subcutaneous injection of
microfat. (**b**) Multiple 1-cm-wide
injections of SNIF perpendicular
to the fold. "1–4" refers to the
sequence and injection points used
when injecting the fat in this area.
(**c**) If the fold has not been erased,
an additional intradermal injection
of SNIF is performed

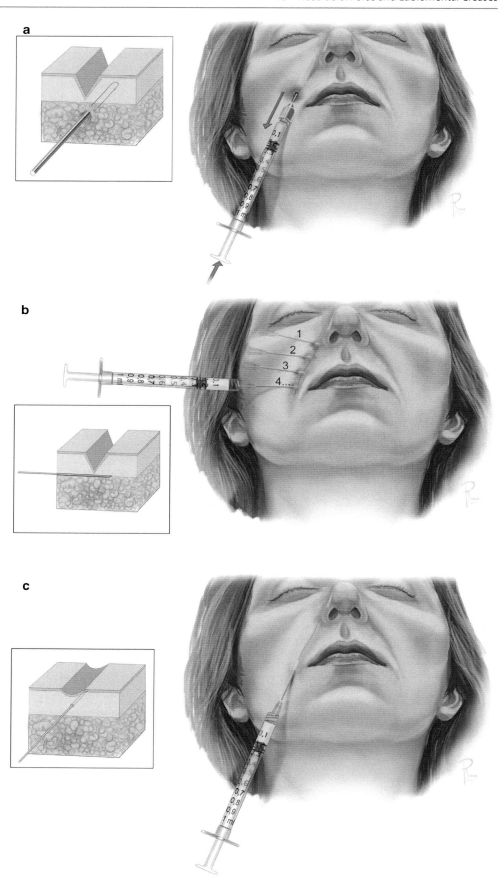

Fig. 10.2 Marionette lines.
(**a**) Subcutaneous injection of
microfat. (**b**) Perpendicular SNIF
injections. "1–3" refers to the
sequence and injection points
used when injecting the fat in this
area

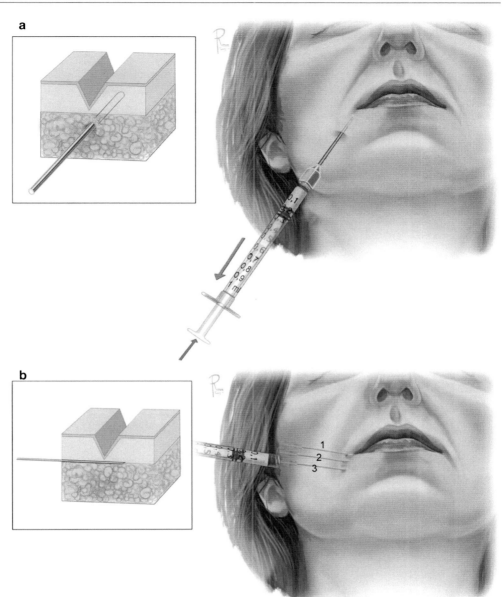

References

1. Rohrich RJ, Ghavami A, Constantine FC, Unger J, Mojallal A. Lift-and-fill face lift: integrating the fat compartments. Plast Reconstr Surg. 2014;133:756e–67.
2. Pezeshk RA, Stark RY, Small KH, Unger JG, Rohrich RJ. Role of autologous fat transfer to the superficial fat compartments for perioral rejuvenation. Plast Reconstr Surg. 2015;136:301e–9.
3. Zeltzer AA, Tonnard PL, Verpaele AM. Sharp-needle intradermal fat grafting (SNIF). Aesthet Surg J. 2012;32:554–61.

Lips and the Perioral Area

11

The lip is an area in which particular care must be taken not to create deformities and overcorrection. We favor performing injections of microfat along the whole of the vermillion border using sharp-needle intradermal fat grafting (SNIF) at a very superficial subcutaneous level because we want the border to appear as a line tracing the whole of Cupid's bow in the upper lip. We use 1 mL of microfat to fill and enhance Cupid's bow (Fig. 11.1a). Then, we perform SNIF in the two philtral columns. We do this subdermally, injecting around 0.5 mL of fat in each column (Fig. 11.1b). This slightly shortens the lip, producing a more youthful appearance.

We then perform the dermal-subdermal filling of the vertical perioral lines. We use microfat for the deeper lines and emulsion (SNIE) for the more superficial ones (Fig. 11.1c). In the lower lip we also make very superficial subcutaneous injections in Cupid's line in the central part of the lip for some 3 mL in the cutaneous mucosa of the vermillion line (Fig. 11.1d). The injection is dermal-subdermal in order to enhance it.

In some cases we perform fat grafting with microfat to fill the lip volume at the level of the muscle [1, 2], but in general we do not favor adding volume to the lips.

© Springer International Publishing Switzerland 2016
J.M. Serra-Renom, J.M. Serra-Mestre, *Atlas of Minimally Invasive Facelift*, DOI 10.1007/978-3-319-33018-1_11

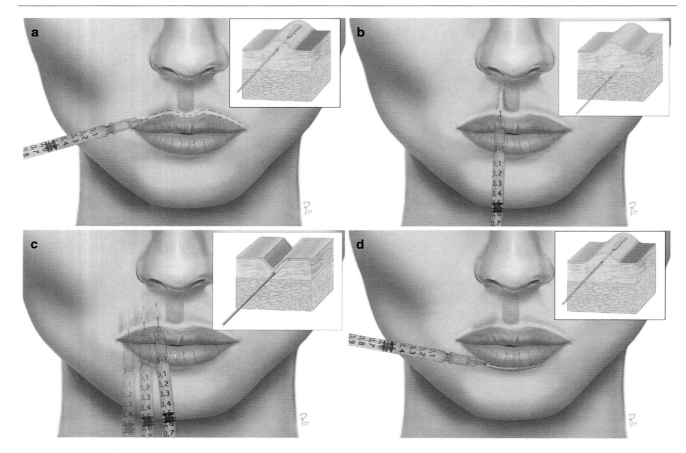

Fig. 11.1 Lips and perioral rejuvenation. (**a**) SNIF in Cupid's bow and in the vermillion border of the upper lip. (**b**) SNIF in the two philtral columns. (**c**) Microfat for the deep perioral lines and/or emulsion in the superficial ones. (**d**) SNIF in the vermillion border of the lower lip

References

1. Gatti JE. Permanent lip augmentation with serial fat grafting. Ann Plast Surg. 1999;42:376–80.
2. Segall L, Ellis DA. Therapeutic options for lip augmentation. Facial Plast Surg Clin North Am. 2007;15:485–90.

Mentoplasty and Mandibular Area

In this chapter we describe two applications that have an important impact on the overall aesthetic appearance of the facial profile. The chin is the most prominent structure in the lower third of the face. Fat grafting in this area represents a simple tool for achieving projection in patients who need minor or moderate correction as well as in those who are unwilling to undergo interventions with alloplastic materials or other techniques but wish to improve this area. The fat technique described in this chapter is a good complement to a rhinoplasty performed in order to harmonize the facial profile. With regard to the prejowls, although the facelift achieves a major correction, injection of fat in this area not only improves outcomes but also helps prevent volume depletions after surgery and delays their reappearance [1, 2].

© Springer International Publishing Switzerland 2016
J.M. Serra-Renom, J.M. Serra-Mestre, *Atlas of Minimally Invasive Facelift*, DOI 10.1007/978-3-319-33018-1_12

12.1   Mentoplasty

This fat grafting technique may or may not be associated with rhinoplasty. When it is associated with rhinoplasty, the rhinoplasty is performed first to remodel the nasal pyramid. Then, the profile surgery is planned.

If surgery to increase chin projection is required, first the mandibular edge is marked with a line from one side of the chin to the other (Fig. 12.1a). Then we draw a vertical line (Fig. 12.1b) and then a spherical ellipse as symmetrical as possible throughout the area where fat grafting will be performed, bearing in mind the midline (Fig. 12.1c).

We make two entry points with a 14-G Abbocath catheter where a vertical line downward from the oral commissure crosses the horizontal line of the mandibular edge. Then, with a Coleman cannula, we perform deep crisscross fat grafting with microfat (Fig. 12.1d).

Normally 2 or 3 mL of microfat is used on each side to reshape the chin, that is, a total of between 4 and 6 mL of microfat. It is important not to alter the concavity between the lower lip and chin and to project the chin's convexity.

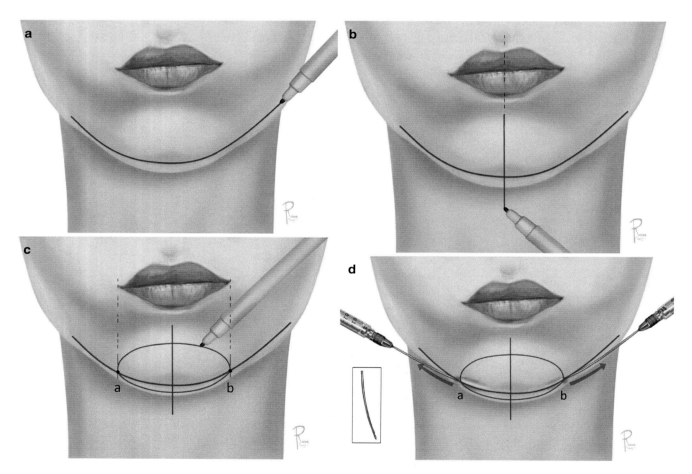

Fig. 12.1 Mentoplasty. Precise markings in this area are important in order to carefully delimit the injection site, as follows. (**a**) A first line marks the mandibular border. (**b**) The central vertical line then divides the chin into two symmetrical parts. (**c**) As indicated in the illustration, a spherical ellipse is drawn from points *a* to *b* that corresponds approximately to the oral commissures. (**d**) Microfat grafting is injected from two injection points to crisscross the grafts

12.2 Lateral Mandibular Ridge Resorption

With aging, signs of bone resorption appear in the whole of the facial skeleton and also in the jaw. A notable depression sometimes appears at the sides of the chin and prejowls (Fig. 12.2a). This is corrected by injecting microfat with a cannula, horizontally, on both sides of the chin (Fig. 12.2b, c).

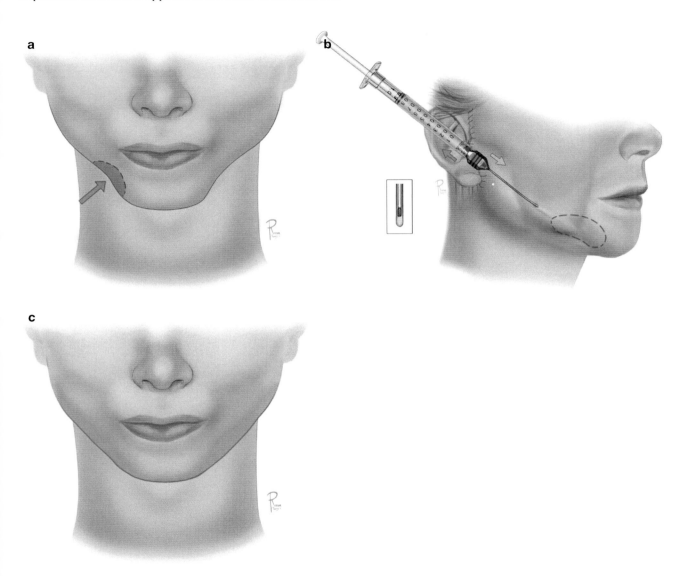

Fig. 12.2 Lipofilling of the lateral mandibular ridge resorption. (**a**) Preoperative view. (**b**) Microfat injection with cannula. (**c**) Correction of the defect

References

1. Metzinger S, Parrish J, Guerra A, Zeph R. Autologous fat grafting to the lower one-third of the face. Facial Plast Surg. 2012;28:21–33.
2. Endara MR, Allred LJ, Han KD, Baker SB. Applications of fat grafting in facial aesthetic skeletal surgery. Aesthet Surg J. 2014;34:363–73.

Nasal Lipofilling

13

It is very important to conduct a thorough medical history in order to determine our objectives in performing subcutaneous fat grafting in any area of the nasal pyramid.

In secondary rhinoplasty this technique is particularly useful [1, 2]. If there is a lateral depression, we mark exactly where we want to perform the fat grafting; if it is a central depression, we define exactly the place where we want to proceed, and if it is throughout the nasal dorsum, we also define it in order to know exactly where to perform the fat grafting.

Once we have finished planning, we disinfect the nasal cavities and the nostrils. With an Abbocath catheter, we make an entry point in the plica nasi between the triangular and the alar cartilages (Fig. 13.1a). If only one side of the nose is to be treated, for a lateral depression, we enter the half of the plica nasi on that side; if we aim to treat the entire the nasal dorsum, we make two entry points in the most medial sites of both plica nasi.

After making the orifices, we introduce the Coleman cannula up to the point we want to reach and then withdraw it longitudinally to fill the defect. The cannula must be introduced atraumatically so as not to perforate the skin. The quantities used are very small: 1–2 cm microfat (Fig. 13.1b).

If there is a depression or scar adhesion, after finishing the injection of microfat, we perform external injections of emulsion in the dermis and in the adhesion (Fig. 13.1c).

© Springer International Publishing Switzerland 2016
J.M. Serra-Renom, J.M. Serra-Mestre, *Atlas of Minimally Invasive Facelift*, DOI 10.1007/978-3-319-33018-1_13

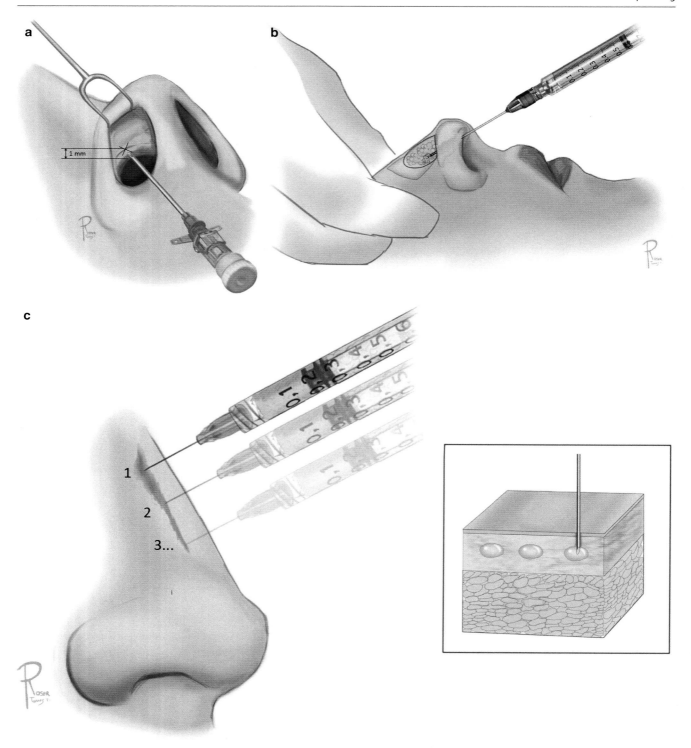

Fig. 13.1 Nasal pyramid. (**a**) Entry point in the plica nasi with an Abbocath. (**b**) Injection of microfat grafting to correct the defect. (**c**) An additional emulsion injection with sharp needle (SNIE) is also performed if there is also a depression or scar retraction. "1–3"refers to the entry points used when injecting the fat

References

1. Baptista C, Nguyen PS, Desouches C, Magalon G, Bardot J, Casanova D. Correction of sequelae of rhinoplasty by lipofilling. J Plast Reconstr Aesthet Surg. 2013;66:805–11.
2. Bénateau H, Rocha CS, Rocha Fde S, Veyssiere A. Treatment of the nasal abnormalities of Hallermann-Streiff syndrome by lipofilling. Int J Oral Maxillofac Surg. 2015;44:1246–9.

14

Neck or Cervical Lipofilling

We treat cervical horizontal wrinkles subdermally with microfat and intrasubdermally with sharp-needle intradermal fat grafting (SNIF), making injections throughout the length of the wrinkle. We proceed very carefully to avoid damaging the vessels because this is a danger zone. We always aspirate before the injection (Fig. 14.1).

© Springer International Publishing Switzerland 2016
J.M. Serra-Renom, J.M. Serra-Mestre, *Atlas of Minimally Invasive Facelift*, DOI 10.1007/978-3-319-33018-1_14

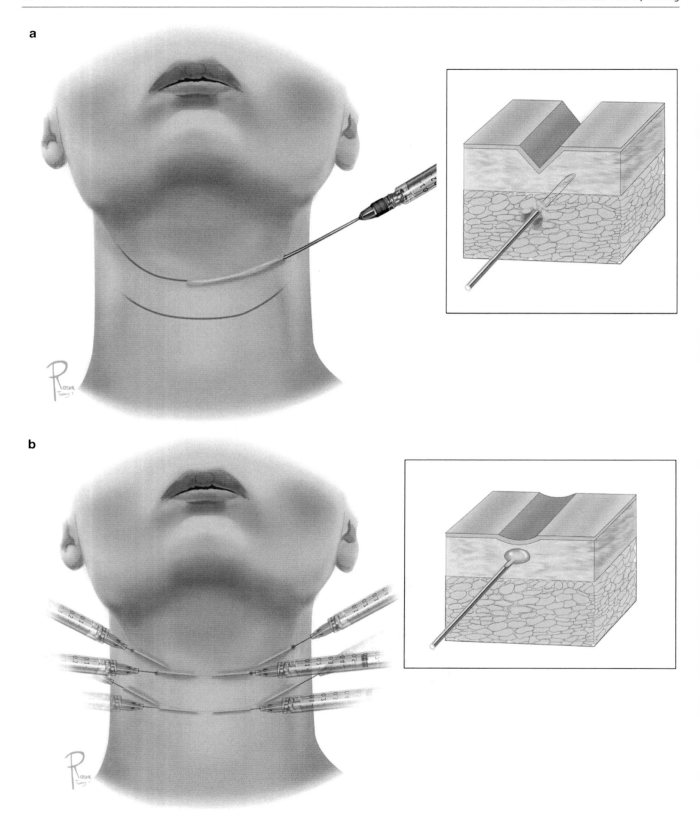

Fig. 14.1 Neck and cervical wrinkles correction. (**a**) Superficial subcutaneous microfat grafting with cannula. (**b**) Intradermal SNIF injection with microfat or emulsion (SNIE)

Facial Mesotherapy

15

Facial mesotherapy is a technique used to rejuvenate the skin by means of intradermal or transdermal injections of variable diluted agents such as multivitamin solutions, homeopathic agents, and other bioactive substances that are thought to improve the signs of skin aging [1].

The good results obtained with fat injection for skin regeneration in cases of cancer surgery after radiotherapy [2–4] extended the applications of fat and the stromal vascular fraction to the area of skin rejuvenation. In recent years we have carried out studies both in the facial region and in the rejuvenation of hands and have achieved significant improvements in skin quality [5–9].

Although the precise role of fat or some of its components in skin rejuvenation is not known, the results suggest an angiogenic action with the formation of new capillaries as well as the reorganization and formation of new elastic fibers in the dermis [6–8].

To perform mesotherapy, we use emulsion, platelet-rich plasma or vitamins either separately or in combination, depending on the needs of each patient. We may only want to perform mesotherapy with emulsion to regenerate and improve the skin, or we may want to use it in combination with platelets to obtain an immediate anti-inflammatory effect if we have performed a facelift and aim to reduce the swelling. We can add vitamins to the emulsion to nourish the dermis, or we might want to use the emulsion with platelets and vitamins. These are the three most frequently used combinations (Fig. 15.1).

Once the most appropriate mix—emulsion + platelets, emulsion + vitamins, and emulsion + platelets + vitamins—has been chosen, we draw the tension columns throughout the cheek in the shape of a curved fan from the zygomatic arch downward toward the nasolabial folds covering the entire cheekbone and then from this point upward throughout the temporal region toward the temporalis crest (Fig. 15.2).

This can also be done in the forehead or in any facial region in which we want to nourish the facial skin. With a 23-G needle, we inject the emulsion mixture following these divergent lines at half-centimeter intervals and in the dermis 2 mm apart, each with a small droplet of the preparation. At the end we apply ointment or oil or cream to soothe the treated region, for example, rosehip oil or a preparation of aloe vera cream. Cold packs may also be useful. If the mesotherapy is part of another treatment and the patient is already sedated, no other anesthetic is required. If it is performed on an outpatient basis, prior application of a topical anesthetic and locoregional block of the infraorbital and temporal nerves are necessary.

© Springer International Publishing Switzerland 2016
J.M. Serra-Renom, J.M. Serra-Mestre, *Atlas of Minimally Invasive Facelift*, DOI 10.1007/978-3-319-33018-1_15

Fig. 15.1 Possible combinations for facial mesotherapy: emulsion (*A*), platelet-rich plasma (*B*), vitamins (*C*)

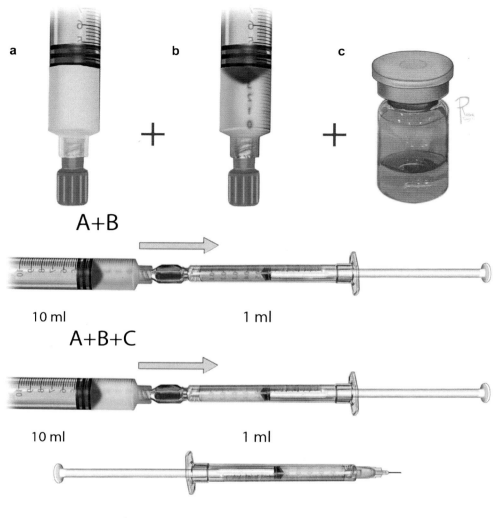

Fig. 15.2 Example of one of the most frequent distributions of injection sites for facial mesotherapy

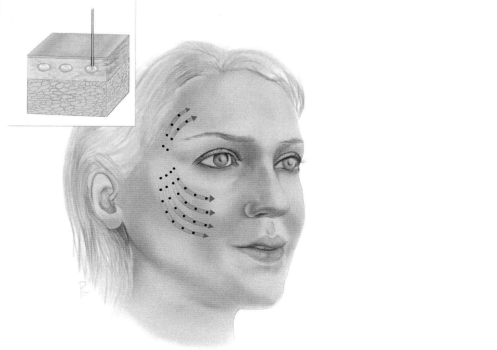

References

1. Atiyeh BS, Ibrahim AE, Dibo SA. Cosmetic mesotherapy: between scientific evidence, science fiction, and lucrative business. Aesthetic Plast Surg. 2008;32:842–9.

2. Rigotti G, Marchi A, Galie M, Baroni G, Benati D, Krampera M, et al. Clinical treatment of radiotherapy tissue damage by lipoaspirate transplant: a healing process mediated by adipose-derived adult stem cells. Plast Reconstr Surg. 2007;119:1409–22.

3. Phulpin B, Gangloff P, Tran N, Bravetti P, Merlin JL, Dolivet G. Rehabilitation of irradiated head and neck tissues by autologous fat transplantation. Plast Reconstr Surg. 2009;123:1187–97.

4. Serra-Renom JM, Muñoz-Olmo JL, Serra-Mestre JM. Fat grafting in postmastectomy breast reconstruction with expanders and prostheses in patients who have received radiotherapy: formation of new subcutaneous tissue. Plast Reconstr Surg. 2010;125:12–8.

5. Coleman SR. Structural fat grafting: more than a permanent filler. Plast Reconstr Surg. 2006;118(3 Suppl):108S–20.

6. Jeong JH. Adipose stem cells and skin repair. Curr Stem Cell Res Ther. 2010;5:137–40.

7. Cohen SR, Mailey B. Adipocyte-derived stem and regenerative cells in facial rejuvenation. Clin Plast Surg. 2012;39:453–64.

8. Charles-de-Sá L, Gontijo-de-Amorim NF, Maeda Takiya C, Borojevic R, Benati D, Bernardi P, et al. Antiaging treatment of the facial skin by fat graft and adipose-derived stem cells. Plast Reconstr Surg. 2015;135:999–1009.

9. Villanueva NL, Hill SM, Small KH, Rohrich RJ. Technical refinements in autologous hand rejuvenation. Plast Reconstr Surg. 2015;136:1175–9.

Facelift

16

Our concept of the facelift is based on two main factors. The first is the gravitational component of aging: ligaments stretch, and tissues tend to descend. This effect is particularly visible in the malar and cervical areas [1].

The other important factor is the loss of volume caused by changes and reabsorption of the facial skeleton [2] and atrophy of the facial fat compartments [3]. This, among other changes, means that the orbit becomes larger, the malar area loses content, and the facial structures lose volume. This is termed the volumetric factor.

When using any facelift technique, the surgeon must take account of both these factors: (1) resolve sagging and excess skin but at the same time do not dissect the tissue so much that the volumetric treatment, including fat grafting with microfat, emulsion, sharp-needle intradermal emulsion (SNIE), sharp-needle intradermal fat grafting (SNIF), and nanofat, cannot be performed. (2) It is also important to avoid the telltale signs of extensive facelifts such as scars in the scalp that cause alopecia or the elimination of the sideburn on stretching or bands at the level of the neck. Scars on the hairline should also be avoided, because although we make them as obliquely or atraumatically as possible, they can often be seen. Sometimes they remain sunken or become hypertrophic. At the same time, the ear must not be allowed to tilt forward or the lobe to grow longer because of skin traction. We now describe some of the main lifting techniques that combine these two principles.

16.1 Inferiorly Pedicled Tongue-Shaped Superficial Musculoaponeurotic System (SMAS) Flap Facelift

This technique [4], as described by the authors, shares the rationale and benefits of a lateral SMASectomy [5]. However, instead of discarding the SMAS, it is used to create an inferiorly pedicle-pointing tongue-shaped flap that is transposed to the mastoid to improve the nasolabial fold and jowls and at the same time to enhance neck contouring during facelift surgery.

Another advantage of this technique is that it does not require an extensive dissection of the SMAS; it does not detach it from the cheek, and it preserves vascularization. This avoids a double scar plane and allows the performance of fat grafting in the central area of the face.

16.1.1 Infiltration of the Tumescent Solution

The tumescent solution is infiltrated subcutaneously in the areas in which the skin dissection is performed. It extends over the parotid region or slightly wider, beginning at the root of the ear just above the level of the sideburn without reaching the hairline and extending behind the ear without reaching the hairline as far as the posterior auricular muscle (Fig. 16.1a, b).

After creating tumescence in the cheek, before starting surgery, we also create tumescence around the neck, in the mandibular edge, and throughout the area up to the insertion of the earlobe (Fig. 16.1c). The tumescent solution contains 1:200,000 adrenaline and lidocaine.

16.1.2 Neck Contouring

It is very important to assess the state of the neck at the preoperative stage and to check skin laxity. By visual inspection and palpation, we determine whether there is a subcutaneous fat component. We also assess the anterior and posterior bands of the platysma muscle, asking the patient to perform maneuvers of platysma muscle contraction in order to plan the surgical intervention in the neck (Fig. 16.2a).

After making the diagnosis, the cervical area is dissected without passing beyond the hyoid bone using nonaggressive lipoaspiration and undermining with a 3-mm flat cannula so as not to create irregularities and adhesions in the skin. We also attempt to leave a layer of subcutaneous fat attached to the skin.

© Springer International Publishing Switzerland 2016
J.M. Serra-Renom, J.M. Serra-Mestre, *Atlas of Minimally Invasive Facelift*, DOI 10.1007/978-3-319-33018-1_16

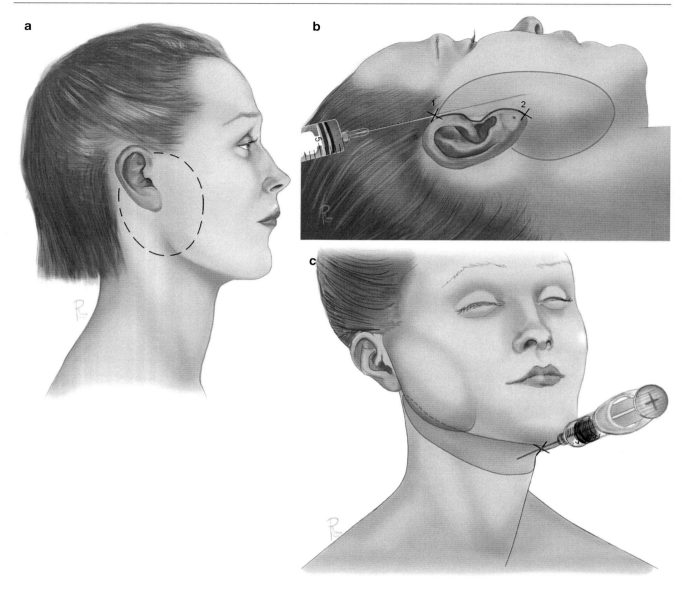

Fig. 16.1 Infiltration of the tumescent solution. (**a**) The area of skin undermining in the cheek and behind the ear. (**b**) Entry points of the needle to create the tumescence in the preauricular area. (**c**) Tumescence is also performed around the neck, in the mandibular edge, and through-

out the area up to the insertion of the earlobe. "1 and 2" represents as said in the figure legend the "Entry points of the needle to create the tumescence in the preauricular area"

This maneuver can be performed without difficulty via three entry points: one at the level of the submental fold and two at the level of the insertion of each earlobe (Fig. 16.2b).

Then, if necessary, we treat the platysma muscle, making an incision at the level of the submental fold. The incision is not made in the fold itself but 2 mm away from it, so that the scar remains hidden and does not appear at the sides when the skin is stretched (Fig. 16.2c).

Then, with the help of a retractor with cold light, the entire subcutaneous plane is dissected with facelift scissors

(Fig. 16.2d). We perform this subcutaneous and supraplatysmal dissection in a triangle, detaching the anterior edges and the two bands of the platysma, reaching the hyoid bone (Fig. 16.2e).

At the level of the hyoid bone, two 2-cm sections are performed on either side so that when the two bands of the platysma muscle are sutured at the midline, there is no redundancy (Fig. 16.2f). Four or five suture stitches are used when midline plication is performed; we never resect the bands because they may adhere to the skin and produce a highly unaesthetic result.

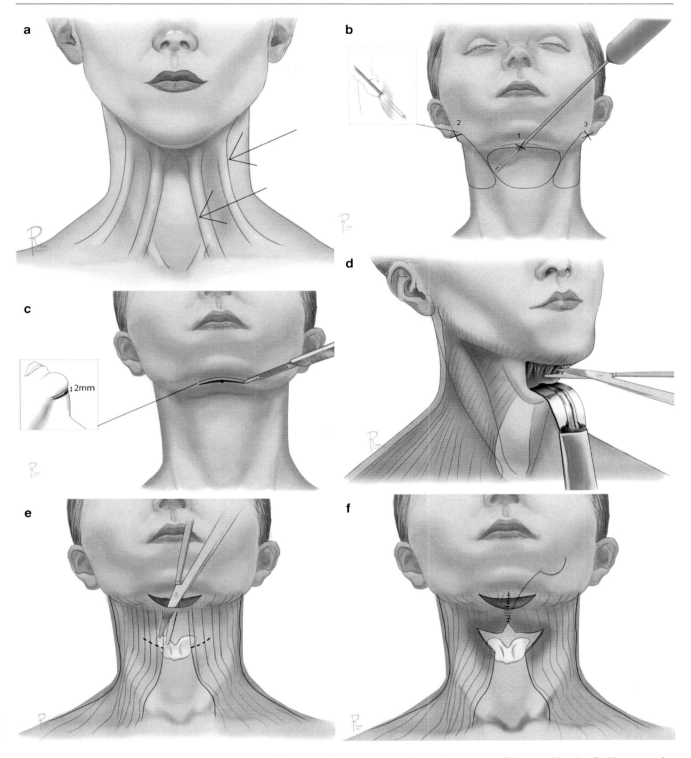

Fig. 16.2 Neck contouring. (**a**) Preoperative analysis of the cervical area. *Arrows* indicate the presence of platysmal bands. (**b**) Nonaggressive lipoaspiration of the neck and jowls. "1–3" represents the entry point trough which liposuction of the neck is performed. (**c**) Submental incision. (**d**) Subcutaneous dissection. (**e**) Myotomy at the hyoid level. (**f**) Midline plication is performed after myotomy at the hyoid level

16.1.3 Skin Undermining

The preauricular incision starts at the highest point of the ear. It continues just 1 mm behind the upper edge of the tragus and then follows the contour down to the lobe (Fig. 16.3a, b).

Then, beneath the skin, leaving a little adipose tissue in the skin flap, we dissect the whole of the marked area with a scalpel or with facelift scissors (Fig. 16.3c, d). This

dissection is performed up to and beyond the edge of the parotid gland. If necessary, the dissection can be extended slightly with the aid of a cold light retractor (Fig. 16.3e).

We then bend the ear forward and mark the retroauricular incision. This incision is not placed exactly on the retroauricular fold but 0.5 cm higher, so that when the skin is stretched, the scar is not visible and remains hidden behind the ear (Fig. 16.3f).

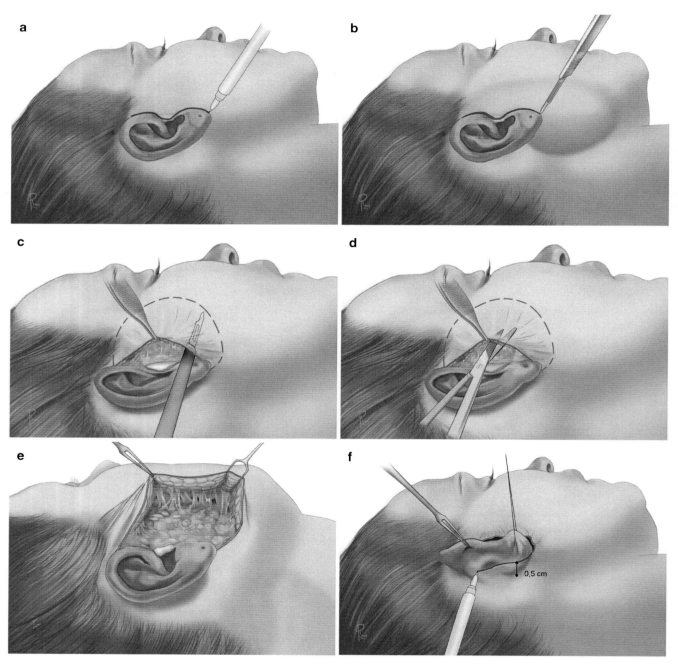

Fig. 16.3 Skin undermining. (**a**) Markings. (**b**) Preauricular incision. (**c**) Subcutaneous dissection over the SMAS can be performed with a scalpel or facelift scissors (**d**). (**e**) Exposure of the SMAS. (**f**) Retroauricular markings. (**g**) Infiltration of the retroauricular area. (**h**) Retroauricular incision. (**i**) Subcutaneous dissection. (**j**) Distal subcutaneous dissection. (**k**) When the cutaneous dissection of the retroauricular region terminates, it joins dissection of the cheek

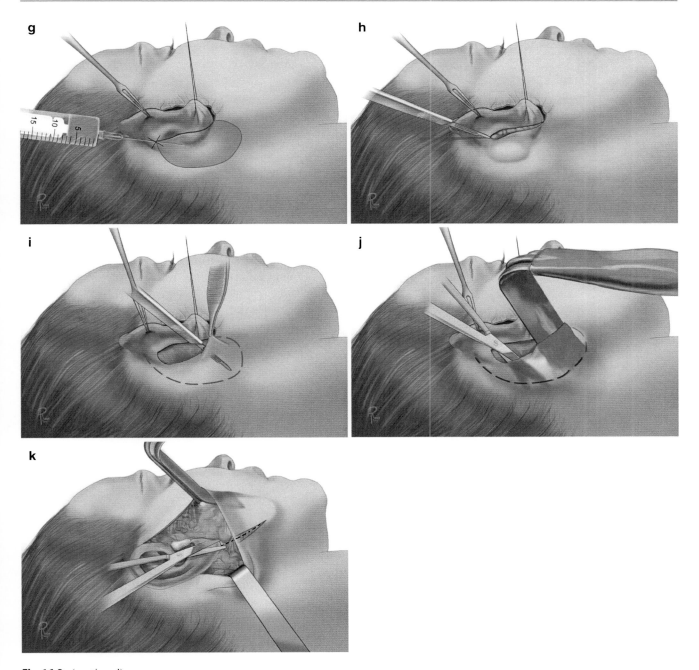

Fig. 16.3 (continued)

The advantage of infiltrating the tumescent solution in this area is that it performs hydrodissection, allowing easy detachment of all the retroauricular skin (Fig. 16.3g). After that, the retroauricular incision is made from the insertion point of the lobe as far as 1 cm above the posterior auricular muscle (Fig. 16.3h).

Dissection of the retroauricular skin is performed with a scalpel or facelift scissors with the aid of a cold light retractor (Fig. 16.3i, j). After this, the preauricular and retroauricular dissections are joined (Fig. 16.3k).

After completing the dissection of the skin flap, rigorous hemostasis is performed with a bipolar coagulator.

16.1.4 SMASplasty

To calculate the size of the SMAS flap, which depends on the flaccidity of the mandibular ridge and nasolabial folds, the pulling test is performed with a forceps (Fig. 16.4a).

After calculating the width of the flap, an oblique tongue-shaped inferiorly pedicled SMAS flap is designed. The inverted U-shaped flap is located approximately 1 cm in front of the lobe and obliquely upward toward the outer edge of the eye, reaching the zygomatic arch and parallel to the nasolabial fold (Fig. 16.4b).

To facilitate the dissection of the flap, it is infiltrated with the tumescent solution described earlier (Fig. 16.4c). It is then dissected from cephalic to caudal up to 1 or 2 cm below the mandibular angle, bearing in mind that we are above the parotid gland but visualizing it clearly and if possible not opening the parotid aponeurosis (Fig. 16.4d).

The flap donor site is closed with a 4-0 continuous absorbable suture (Fig. 16.4e). In this way the nasolabial fold and the mandibular edge are corrected. After that the SMAS is rotated, stretched, and sutured with a 3-0 absorbable suture

at several points at the height of the mastoid (Fig. 16.4f). With this traction, the neck adapts very well, and the angle of the jaw is also correct.

Once the flap has been sutured, we make two or three stitches in the side of the platysma muscle and suture it to the sternocleidomastoid muscle (Fig. 16.4g).

16.1.5 Skin Closure

To apply the traction of the skin flaps in the correct direction and to be able to calculate the amount of skin to be resected, we use two Lahey forceps, one positioned in the upper preauricular area and the other behind the ear.

We pull the preauricular part slightly upward and outward, avoiding any folds or excess areas in the upper edge of the wound, and move the retroauricular area vertically in an upward direction, finding a position that allows us a proper adaptation of the skin (Fig. 16.5a).

Two parallel sections of the skin flap are performed until the upper and lower edges of the tragus are seen; there we

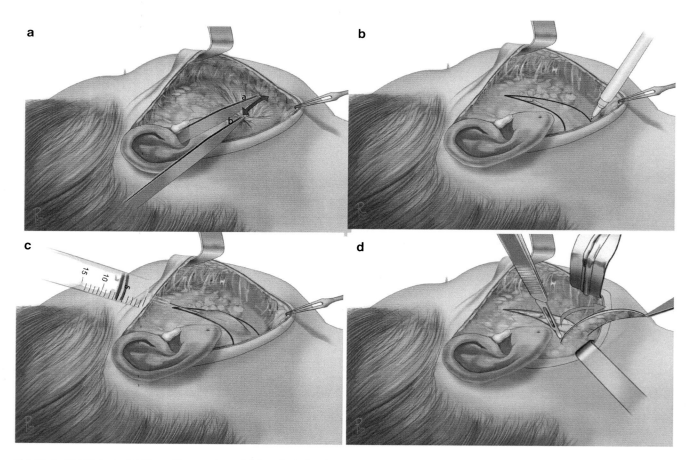

Fig. 16.4 SMASplasty. (**a**) The pulling test is useful for calculating the dimensions of the flap. "a" and "b" represents the pulling test of the SMAS from one point to another to assess the quantity of SMAS that will be removed. (**b**) Design of the SMAS flap. (**c**) Infiltration of a tumescent solution. (**d**) Elevation of the flap. (**e**) Closure of the donor site. (**f**) Transposition of the SMAS flap in a posterosuperior direction and secured to the mastoid fascia. (**g**) An additional platysmal plication can be performed with 2 to 4 sutures as indicated with the numbers

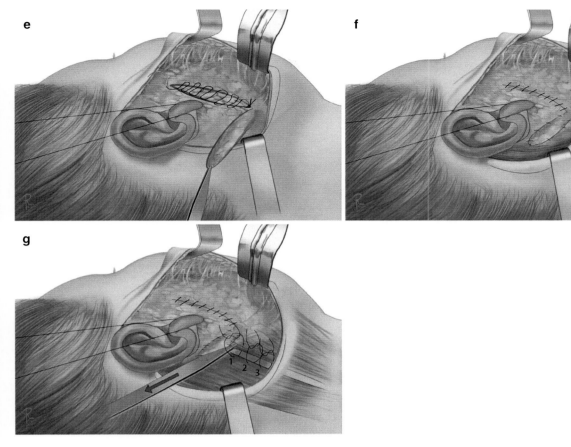

Fig. 16.4   (continued)

attach the cheek skin flap to a fixed structure, the external ear canal, with two U-shaped 3-0 Prolene stitches (Fig. 16.5c, d).

These two stitches in the external ear canal maintain the traction of the flap without deforming or widening the ear canal, allowing us to avoid the necessity of extending the incision as far as the temporal region or hairline, and therefore without altering the line of the sideburn or the hairline at the nape of the neck.

Then the excess skin above and below the tragus is resected, making sure that it is perfectly aligned with the incision previously made in the ear (Fig. 16.5e).

On reaching the lobe, it is very important to resect it without tension. Then, with the section along the lobe already made, in order to prevent tension, we make a subcutaneous stitch in the lobe, enabling its attachment to the deep plane (Fig. 16.5f).

To resect the retroauricular skin, we bend the ear forward, and with moderate traction and ensuring that the lobe does not fold and remains flat, we section it as far as the upper edge of the incision at the position of the posterior auricular muscle (Fig. 16.5g). In the resected area, the wound edges are asymmetrical, much shorter in the ear than in the retroauricular skin flap. This is later corrected with sutures (Fig. 16.5h).

After suturing the back of the lobe without puckering (area b in the illustration) and reaching the level of the concha, we pucker the area with great care (Fig. 16.5i), taking more tissue from the inferior than from the superior border to regularize the wound. We do this with a moderate running suture with very small loops using Vicryl rapide 4-0. From the concha upward, it is very important to make a moderate puckering maneuver taking more tissue from the skin behind the ear than from the skin of the ear itself to be able to obtain tissue and complete the whole of the suture.

At the upper end, it is sometimes necessary to extend the incision a little to correct a small dog ear, but this extension remains within the retroauricular fold. The puckering is not of concern us because within a month it will be fully resolved (Fig. 16.5j).

When suturing the anterior part, it is very important to restructure the tragus particularly well, and for this reason, we proceed with great care. First, at the anterior base of the tragus, we resect a couple of millimeters in the deep layer so that the skin can distribute and penetrate a little in this

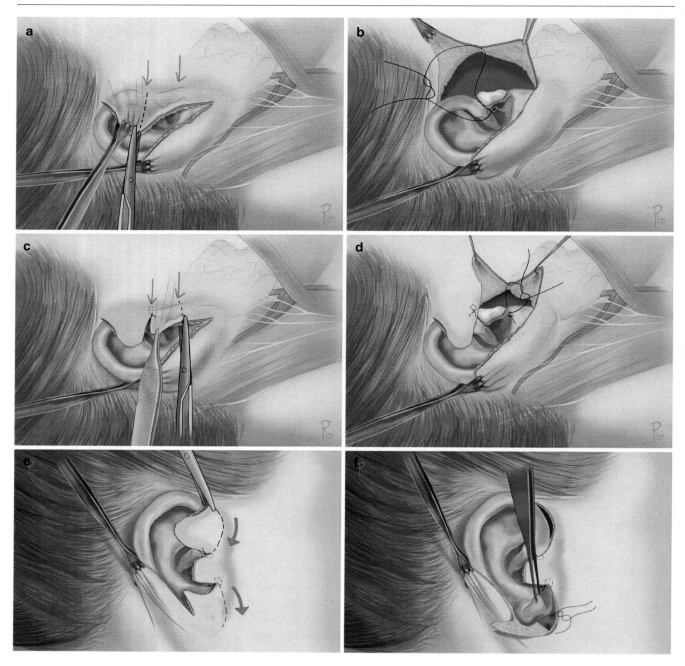

Fig. 16.5 Skin closure. (**a**) Adaptation of the skin without the formation of dog ears at the two ends of the incisions. (**b**) Attachment point of the skin flap to the external auditory canal. (**c**) Section of the skin flap until we see the lower edge of the tragus. (**d**) Second attachment point of the skin flap to the external auditory canal. (**e**) Resection of the excess skin above and below the tragus. (**f**) Subcutaneous stitch in the lobe in order to attach it to the deep plane. (**g**) Resection of the excess skin. (**h**) Asymmetry between the edges of the retroauricular wound, which must be corrected with sutures. (**i**) After suturing the back of the lobe and reaching the concha (zone a), we perform a suture, wrinkling the skin (zone b). (**j**) Retroauricular skin closure. (**k**) Resection of a portion of the deep layer in the pretragal area. (**l**) Defatting the tragus flap. (**m**) Tragus reconstruction. (**n**) Completion of the skin closure. (**o**) Correction of the facial negative vector with fat grafting. "1–4" indicates the multiple passes when injecting the fat in order to creat a criss-cross pattern of injection. (**p**) Injection of activated platelet-rich plasma

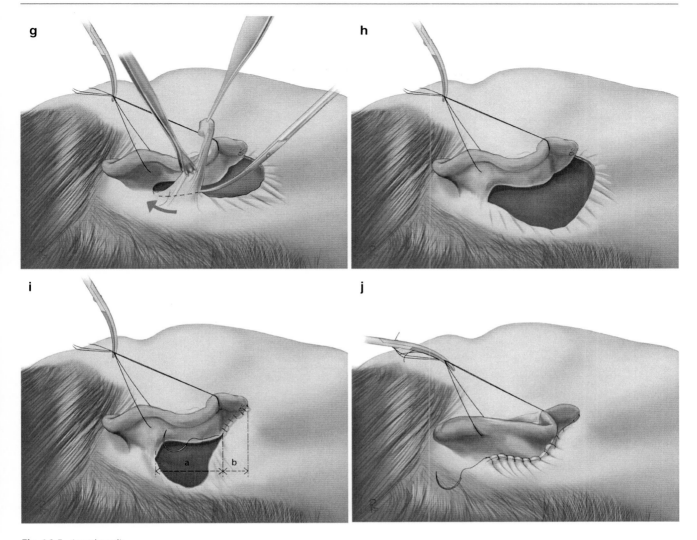

Fig. 16.5   (continued)

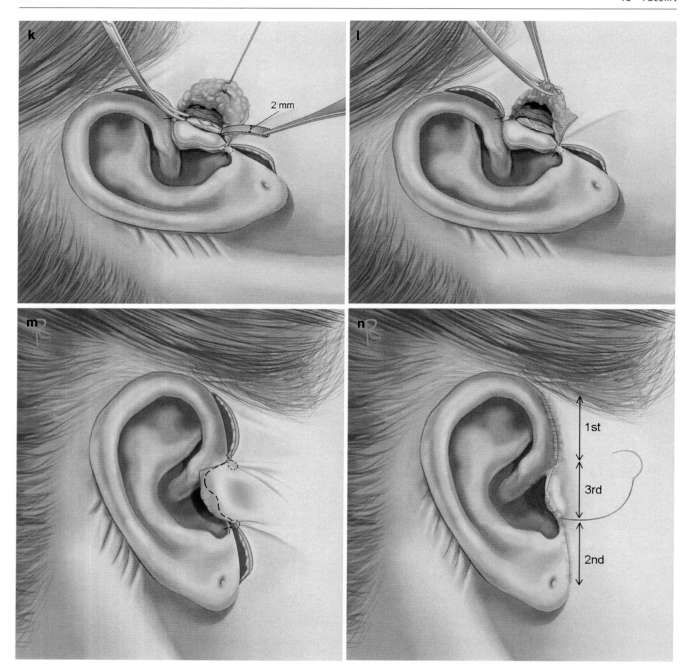

Fig. 16.5 (continued)

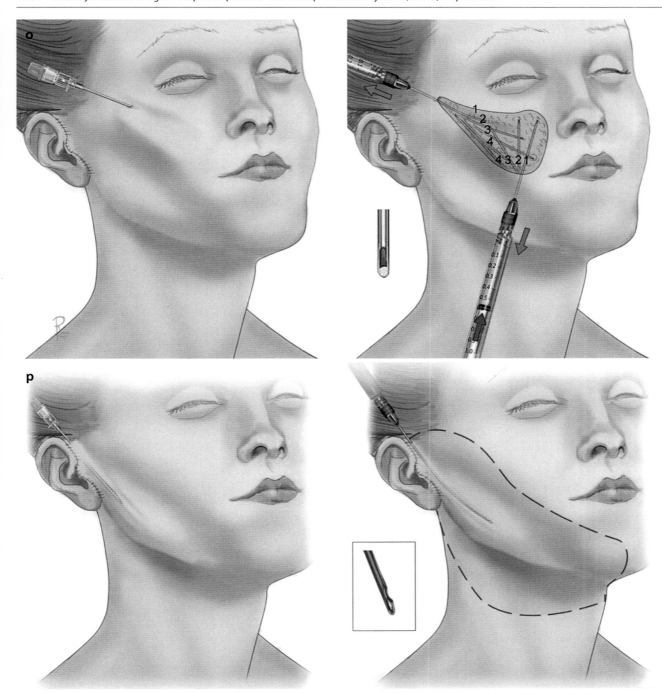

Fig. 16.5 (continued)

pretragal area and mask the effect of the facelift (Fig. 16.5k). Then, we evert the skin at the level of the tragus and remove the fat so that the skin will remodel well and fit the tragus perfectly (Fig. 16.5l).

When we have emptied the pretragal area and have thinned the skin of the tragus, we make a suture without tension and with substantial amounts of tissue to achieve an aesthetically pleasing effect in the tragus. It is very important that both tragi are identical, contoured, and not too small. We then suture the skin to the tragus (Fig. 16.5m) and complete the suturing of the preauricular incision. This suture is performed with a 5-0 monofilament nylon in a running or intradermal fashion (Fig. 16.5n).

Once the surgery is complete, fat grafting in the malar area is performed in order to optimize the symmetry of both hemifaces, correct the negative vector, and restore the facial contour [6] (Fig. 16.5o). At this point, and depending on the needs of each patient, we perform the other facial fat grafting techniques described in the previous chapters.

Subsequently, with a 1-mm blunt cannula, we inject activated platelet-rich plasma (PRP) in the whole of the dissected area (Fig. 16.5p). In our experience, the injection of PRP associated with lifting limits the inflammation and reduces the ecchymosis and postoperative drainage at 24 h.

We leave two drains in place, without aspiration. The drain is placed with a needle in the scalp, but we keep it closed without aspiration for 4 h. Also, in the first 24 h, a compressive cervicofacial bandage is applied with a layer of sponge across the cervical area to above the ear; the sponge is dynamic, keeping the tissue active and preventing the formation of hematomas.

16.2 SMAS Plication

Besides the technique described above based on an inverted U-shaped SMAS flap, other minimally invasive procedures can be performed. A very useful one is SMAS plications [7].

Basically, the subcutaneous dissection is the same as in most minimally invasive facelifts. After performing the pinch test to decide on the plication (or plications) to per-

form, without undermining the SMAS, we pucker it and suture it to its new position (Fig. 16.6a, b).

SMAS plications are fast, simple to perform, and safe, but they may cause bulging in the puckered area (Fig. 16.6c).

In this way we do not have to detach the SMAS, and we have not risked facial nerve injury, although there is a small bulge in the puckered area. In some cases this procedure is indicated (Fig. 16.6d).

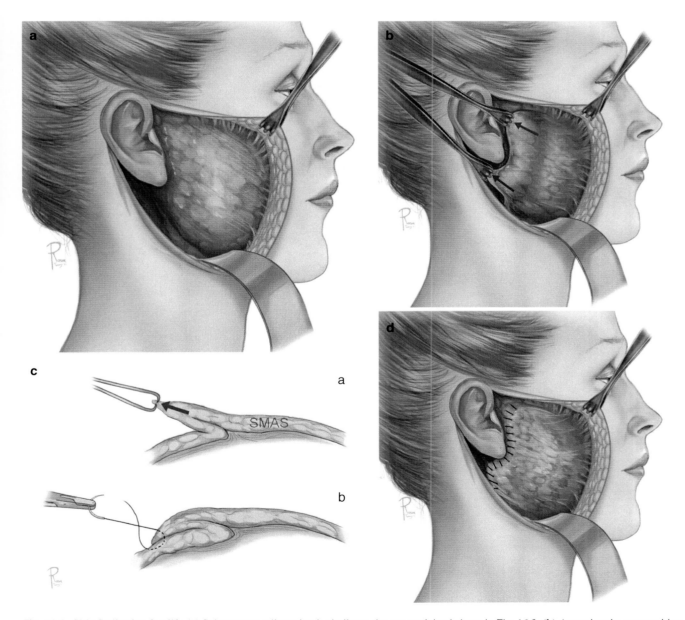

Fig. 16.6 SMAS plication facelift. (**a**) Subcutaneous dissection is similar to the one explained above in Fig. 16.3. (**b**) Assessing the new position of the SMAS. *Arrows* represents the vector or direction of traction of the SMAS. (**c**) Performance of the plication: "a" plication of the SMAS, "b" suture it to its new position. (**d**) One or more plications can be performed. This is one of the most frequently used plications

16.3   SMASectomy

The SMASectomy, first described by Baker [5, 8], consists of an oblique resection of an ellipse of the SMAS from the outer edge to the mandibular angle. The defect is then sutured and the nasolabial folds corrected. However, the procedure does not correct the neck, and it also makes an incision in front of the sideburn and the hairline (Fig. 16.7).

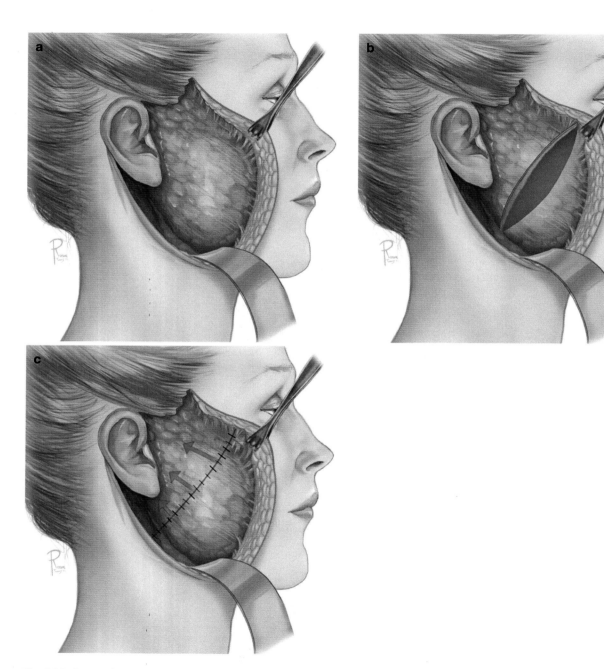

Fig. 16.7 Lateral SMASectomy. (**a**) Exposure of the SMAS. (**b**) An ellipse of the SMAS is excised over the parotid gland. (**c**) An anterior mobile SMAS, which is not separated from the deeper planes and thus maintains its vascularization and elasticity, is advanced and sutured to the posterior SMAS fixed by the retaining ligaments

16.4 MACS Facelift (Minimal Access Cranial Suspension)

Tonnard and coworker [9] described both the simple and the extended forms of the MACS facelift.

An inverted L-shaped cutaneous incision is performed from the base of the ear lobe, passing in front of the ear and until the inferior limit of the sideburn. In the extended version, the incision continues along the anterior border of the temporal hairline.

Skin dissection is only subcutaneous, running from 1 cm above the zygomatic arch to the mandibular angle and about 5 cm in the anterior direction. Two U-shaped purse-string sutures are performed with 2-0 Prolene on the nonundermined superficial musculoaponeurotic system, with anchoring to the deep temporal fasciae (Fig. 16.8).

The extended MACS lift not only lengthens the cutaneous incision but also extends the subcutaneous undermining over the area of the malar fat pad; this makes it possible to perform a third purse-string suture between the deep temporal fasciae and the malar fat pad.

Although we do not favor the preauricular incision, the results obtained with this technique are also very satisfactory.

References

1. Furnas DW. The retaining ligaments of the cheek. Plast Reconstr Surg. 1989;83:11–6.
2. Mendelson B, Wong CH. Changes in the facial skeleton with aging: implications and clinical applications in facial rejuvenation. Aesthetic Plast Surg. 2012;36:753–60.
3. Rohrich RJ, Pessa JE. The fat compartments of the face: anatomy and clinical implications for cosmetic surgery. Plast Reconstr Surg. 2007;119:2219–27. Discussion 2228–31.
4. Serra-Renom JM, Diéguez JM, Yoon T. Inferiorly pedicled tongue-shaped SMAS flap transposed to the mastoid to improve the nasolabial fold and jowls and enhance neck contouring during face-lift surgery. Plast Reconstr Surg. 2008;121:298–304.
5. Baker DC. Lateral SMASectomy. Plast Reconstr Surg. 1997;100:509–13.
6. Serra-Renom JM, Serra-Mestre JM. Periorbital rejuvenation to improve the negative vector with blepharoplasty and fat grafting in the malar area. Ophthal Plast Reconstr Surg. 2011;27:442–6.
7. Baker DC. Lateral SMASectomy, plication and short scar facelifts: indications and techniques. Clin Plast Surg. 2008;35:533–50.
8. Baker DC. Minimal incision rhytidectomy (short scar face lift) with lateral SMASectomy. Aesthet Surg J. 2001;21:68–79.
9. Tonnard P, Verpaele A. The MACS-lift short scar rhytidectomy. Aesthet Surg J. 2007;27:188–98.

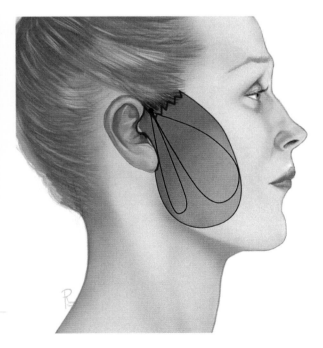

Fig. 16.8 MACS facelift

Clinical Cases

This chapter presents brief histories of several patients who have undergone some of the facial fat grafting techniques described in the previous chapters for correction of volume defects or for fine contouring of superficial wrinkles.

17.1   Clinical Case 1

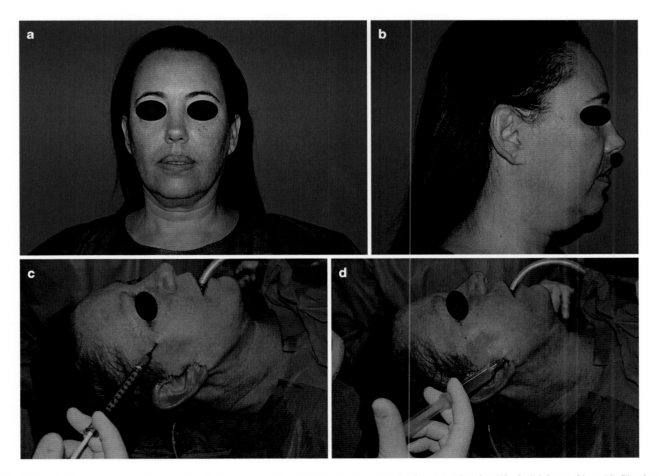

Fig. 17.1 A 55-year-old patient requesting facial rejuvenation. (**a**) Frontal view. (**b**) Profile. (**c**) After facelift: facial fat grafting. (**d**) Platelets throughout the area of the neck dissection. (**e**) Frontal view 1-year postsurgery. (**f**) Side view 1-year postsurgery

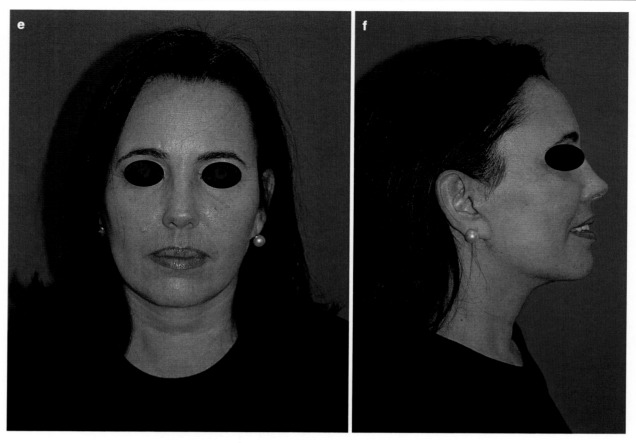

Fig. 17.1 (continued)

17.2   **Clinical Case 2**

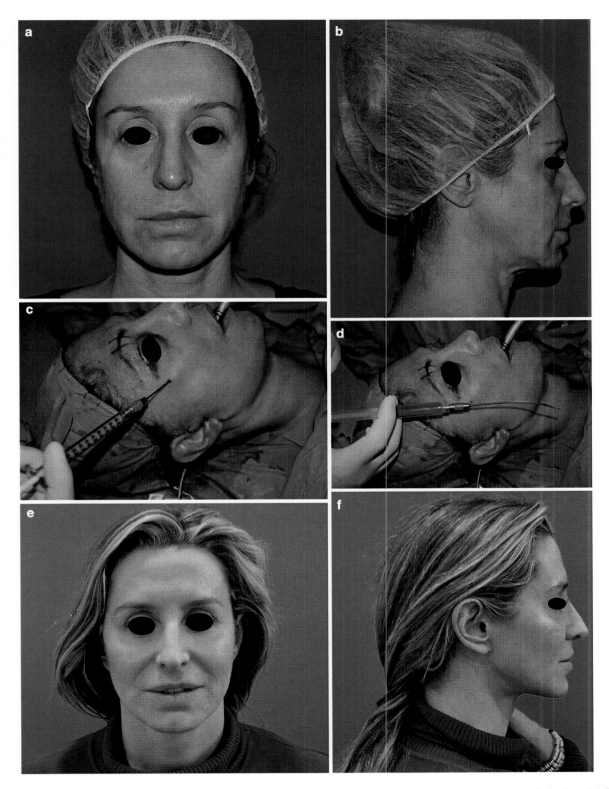

Fig. 17.2 A 45-year-old patient requesting facial rejuvenation. (**a**) Preoperative frontal view. (**b**) Preoperative side view. (**c**) Intraoperative image. After the facelift, fat grafting with microfat was performed in the periorbital and malar areas. (**d**) Injection of platelets. (**e**) Frontal view 1-year postsurgery. (**f**) Side view 1-year postsurgery

17.3   Clinical Case 3

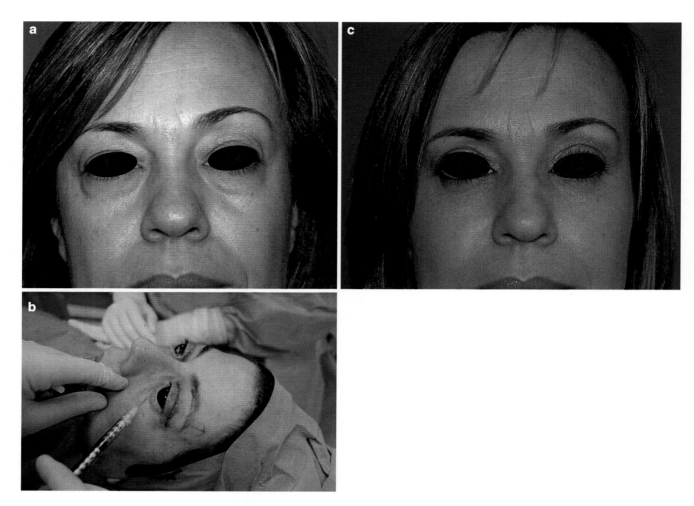

Fig. 17.3 A 60-year-old patient requesting periorbital rejuvenation. (**a**) Preoperative image showing excess skin in the upper eyelid, bags under the eyes, tear trough, and facial negative vector with sinking of the malar fat pad. (**b**) Intraoperative image after performing open upper blepharoplasty, transconjunctival lower blepharoplasty, and fat grafting of the tear trough and the lower lid with emulsion. (**c**) View 1-year postsurgery

17.4   Clinical Case 4

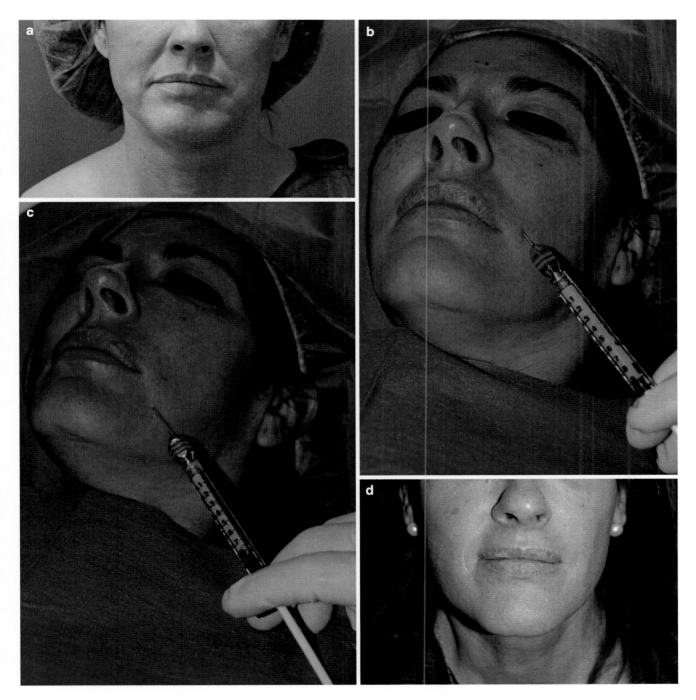

Fig. 17.4 Patient requesting facial rejuvenation with fat grafting alone. (**a**) Frontal preoperative view. (**b**) Microfat in nasolabial folds. (**c**) Microfat in marionette folds. (**d**) View 1-year after fat grafting of the perioral region

17.5   Clinical Case 5

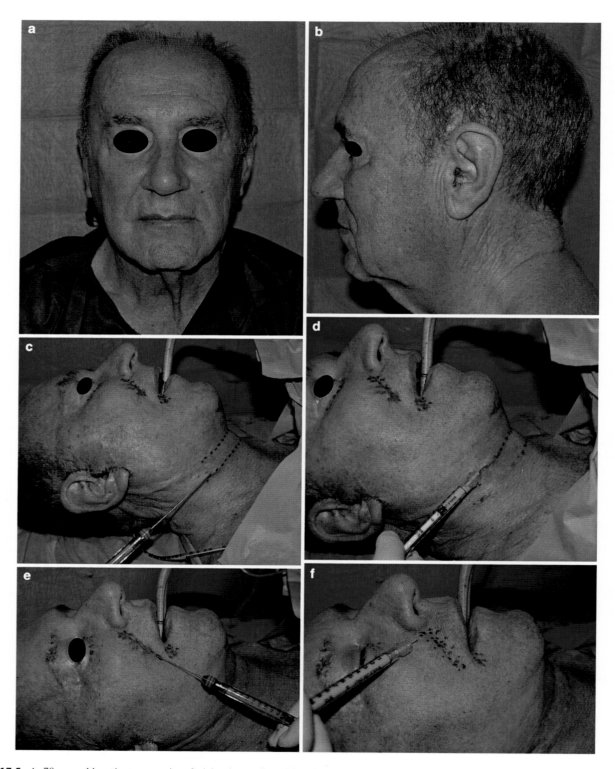

Fig. 17.5 A 70-year-old patient requesting facial rejuvenation. (**a**) Preoperative frontal view. (**b**) Preoperative side view. (**c**) Fat grafting with microfat of cervical wrinkles. (**d**) Sharp-Needle intradermal fat graft (SNIF) of cervical wrinkles. (**e**) Microfat in nasolabial folds. (**f**) Perpendicular injections of SNIF in the nasolabial fold. (**g**) Additional intradermal SNIF injection to remove nasolabial fold wrinkle. (**h**) SNIF to fill marionette folds. (**i**) SNIF perpendicular to marionette folds. (**j**) SNIF and microfat in the eyebrows. (**k**) SNIF in crow's feet. (**l**) Correction of the glabelar area. (**m**) Frontal view 1-year postsurgery. (**n**) Side view 1-year postsurgery

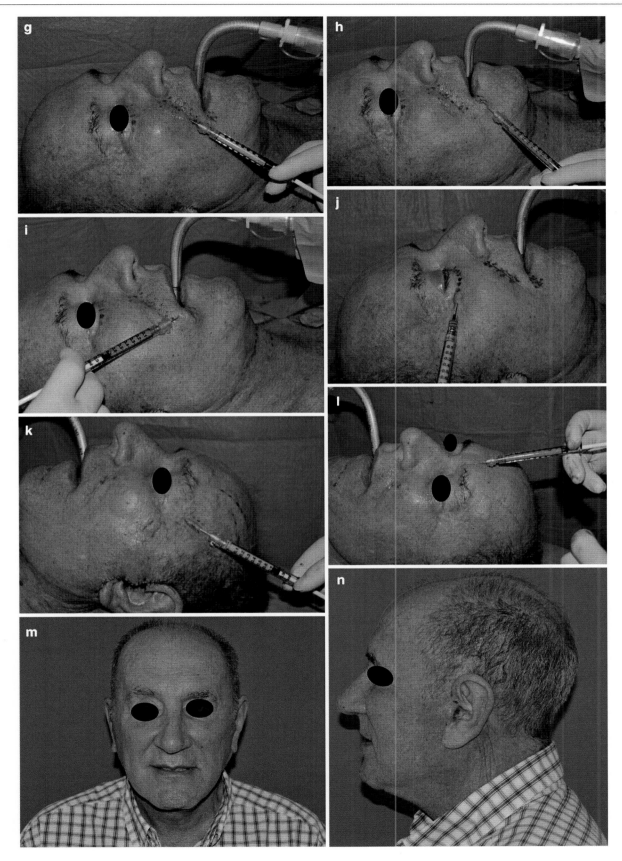

Fig. 17.5 (continued)

17.6   Clinical Case 6

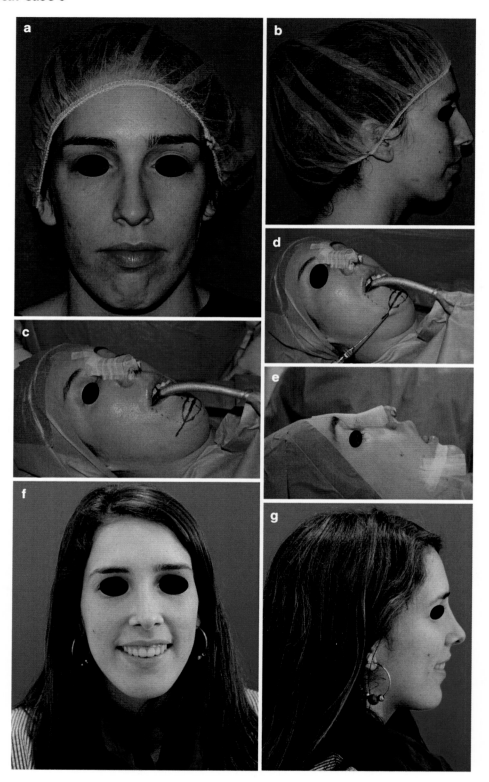

Fig. 17.6 A 20-year-old patient requesting correction of the nasal pyramid. (**a**) Preoperative frontal view. (**b**) Preoperative side view. Assessment of the profile shows chin hypoplasia. (**c**) Rhinoplasty already performed. Design of the area for performing fat grafting of the chin. (**d**) Fat grafting in the chin with microfat using a Coleman cannula. (**e**) Immobilization of the graft in the chin. (**f**) Frontal view 1-year postsurgery. (**g**) Side view showing the harmony achieved with the fat grafting at the level of the chin

17.7 Clinical Case 7

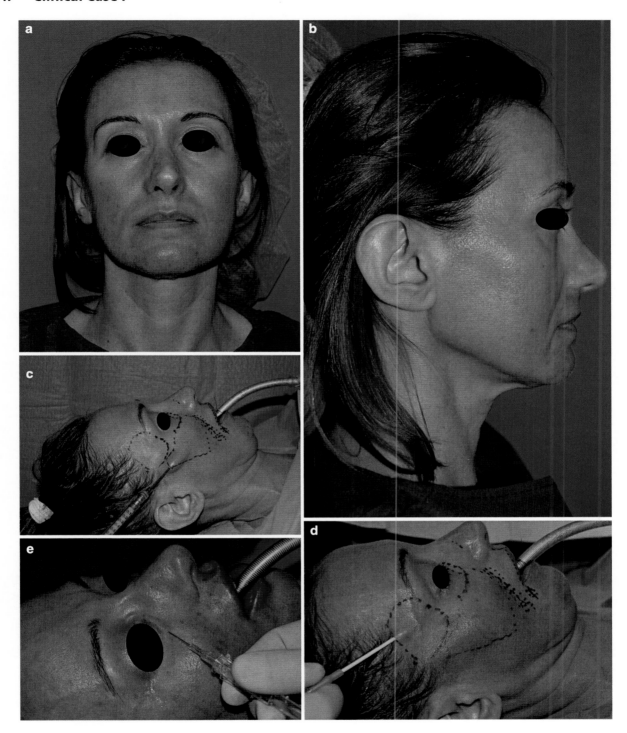

Fig. 17.7 A 39-year-old patient requesting noninvasive facial rejuvenation. Fat grafting performed throughout the facial area. (**a**) Preoperative frontal view. (**b**) Preoperative side view. (**c**) Fat grafting with microfat in the malar region. (**d**) Portal for performing fat grafting in the temporal region. (**e**) Use of an Abbocath 16 (Abbott Ireland Ltd., Sligo, Republic of Ireland) to introduce the cannula for correction of the tear trough. (**f**) Correction of tear trough using a cannula. (**g**) Use of an Abbocath 16 to perform fat grafting in the region of lower eyelid. (**h**) Microfat and emulsion for the lower eyelid with cannula. (**I**) Abbocath to create the portal for correction of crow's feet and the outer edge. (**j**) Cannula for filling the lateral orbital rim and crow's feet. (**k**) SNIF for lengthwise correction of nasolabial folds. (**l**) SNIF for perpendicular correction of nasolabial folds. (**m**) SNIF for lengthwise correction of marionette folds. (**n**) SNIF in the Cupid's bow of the upper lip. (**o**) SNIF in Cupid's line in the lower lip. (**p**) SNIF with microfat to correct philtral columns. (**q**) Mesotherapy with emulsion and platelets. (**r**) View at the end of the intervention. (**s**) Frontal view 1-year postsurgery. (**t**) Oblique view 1-year postsurgery

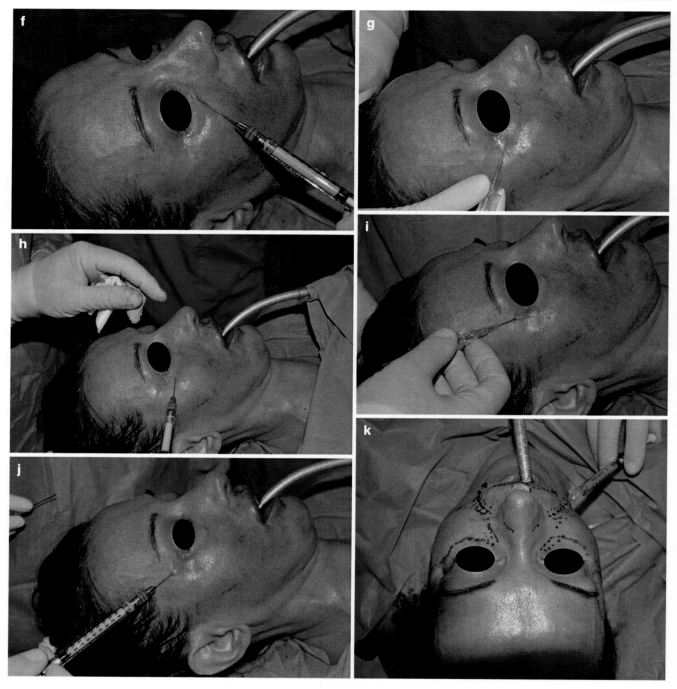

Fig. 17.7 (continued)

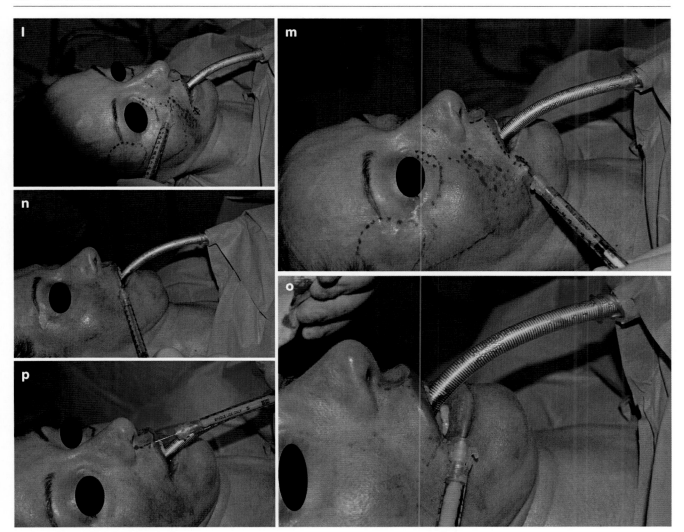

Fig. 17.7 (continued)

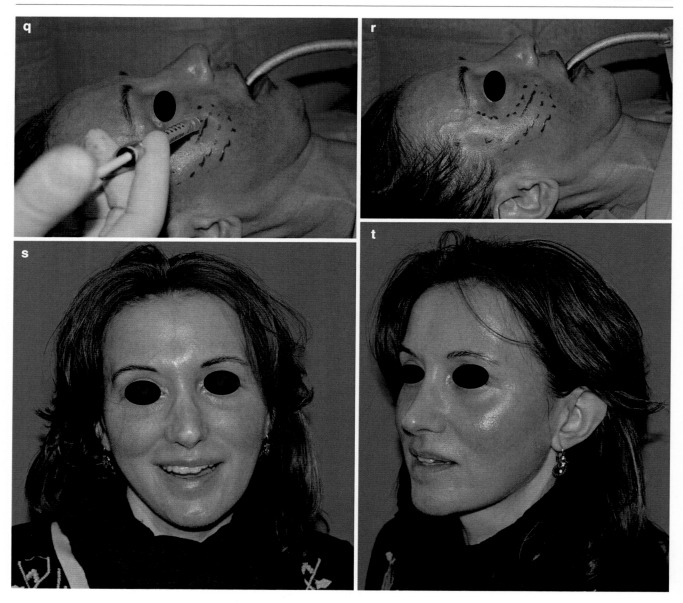

Fig. 17.7 (continued)

17.8   **Clinical Case 8**

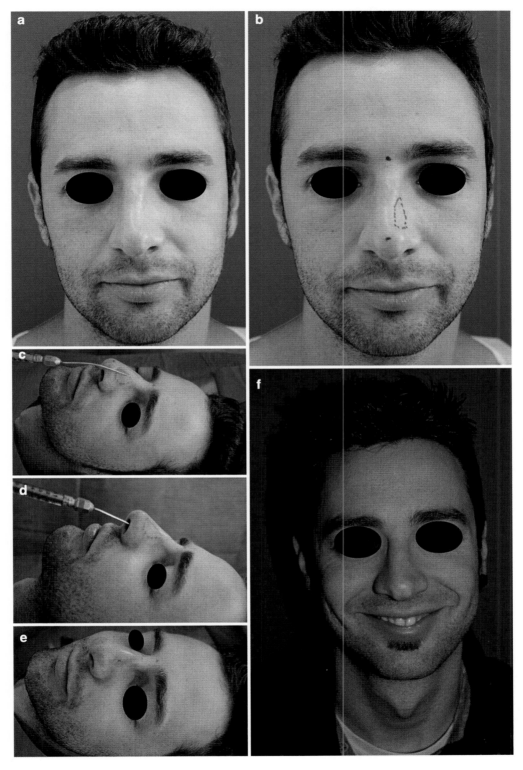

Fig. 17.8 Patient who suffered nasal trauma and presents with deviation and sinking of the left side. Refuses rhinoplasty but seeks improvement. The depression of the left side is filled with microfat. (**a**) Preoperative frontal view. (**b**) Careful design of areas for the fat grafting. (**c**) Microfat introduced downward with a blunt cannula, taking great care not ro pierce the skin of the nasal dorsum. (**d**) Insertion of the cannula via the plica nasi and localization of the edge of the end of the cannula to perform fat grafting. (**e**) Immediate postoperative view after fat grafting. (**f**) View 1-year postsurgery

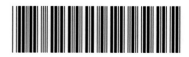